Battling the Killer Within
and Winning

www.battlingthekillerwithin.com

Battling the Killer Within and Winning

Thomas A. Farrington

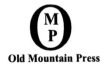

Old Mountain Press

Published by:
Old Mountain Press, Inc.
2542 S. Edgewater Dr.
Fayetteville, NC 28303

www.oldmountainpress.com

ISBN: 1-931575-52-5
Library of Congress Control Number: 2004195484

ProstRcision® is a registered trademark of the Radiotherapy Clinics of Georgia.
Battling the Killer Within and Winning.

First Edition
Manufactured in the United States of America
1 2 3 4 5 6 7 8 9 10

Disclaimer

This book is not intended to be a medical guide (and should not be used as such) for those seeking medical treatment, and medical counseling and support. Doctors and other medical specialists should be consulted when selecting medical treatments.

This book is dedicated to the memories of my father:

Osmond Thomas Farrington Jr.,

My grandfathers:

Osmond Thomas Farrington Sr.

Thomas Wesley Gattis

And

To the hopes of the men who volunteered their stories.

To those survivors active in the "War on prostrate cancer."

Acknowledgments

To Juarez, my wife, who has been by my side throughout this battle with prostate cancer, and an invaluable asset to me while writing this book. I say thank you an infinite number of times. Your love and compassion have been my strength. God has truly blessed me with your presence.

Thanks to my children, Christopher, Trevor, and Tomeeka, whose support, love and care have been uplifting, and invaluable in helping me establish the Prostate Health Education Network (PHEN).

My mother, Mary Farrington, and sister, Geraldine Martin, have been a blessing in helping me face my health crisis. Thank you for everything.

Sharon Deyett, my administrative assistant, worked with me in preparing the many manuscript drafts, and was a constant source of support and encouragement throughout all my challenges. Thank you.

Thanks to my pastor, Rev. Dr. Larry Edmunds and my St. John's Baptist Church family for your many prayers. They make a difference.

To my many friends in Boston, Atlanta, and around the country, my deepest appreciation for your support, thoughtfulness, telephone calls and prayers.

Thanks to Radiotherapy Clinics of Georgia for a comprehensive treatment program and for teaching me about prostate cancer.

To the Atlanta Hope Lodge, thanks for being there.

Sincere appreciations to the Dana - Farber Cancer Institute, the Massachusetts Prostate Cancer Coalition and the National Black Leadership Initiative on Cancer (NBLIC) for their support of the Prostate Health Education Network, Inc. (PHEN) programs.

Darla Bruno performed the final editing for this book.

Contents

Message to the Reader

In 2005, I celebrate five years as a prostate cancer survivor. While I was in treatment in the year 2000, I began writing a book about my experience and the experiences of nineteen men in treatment with me. I thought our stories could be helpful to other men facing prostate cancer. The resultant book, *Battling the Killer Within* was released in 2001. The book has been nationally acclaimed and quite successful in meeting my goals. It has served the needs of thousands of men and enabled me to become very active in the War on Prostate Cancer.

In 2004, I recognized a need to enhance and update *Battling the Killer Within*; in doing so, I also changed the title. *Battling the Killer Within and Winning* contains a new chapter entitled, "Winning," two additional appendices, and updated data. *Battling the Killer Within and Winning* provides an increased focus on the psychological aspects of beating prostate cancer. It also emphasizes prostate health awareness and contains an important guide to help all men understand and manage their prostate health.

Prostate cancer probably touches every family in the Unites States at some level, and many other families around the world. The word cancer brings fear and a sense of hopelessness to many of whom it touches.

When I was diagnosed with prostate cancer, I endured all of the shock and fear associated with the big "C." Because of my family history with this cancer, I knew it was a relentless killer. This perhaps led to an increased level of fear that caused me to make a treatment decision that I reversed at the last moment.

I eventually chose a treatment that led me to spend seven weeks in Atlanta, Georgia, away from my home in Concord, Massachusetts. This turned out to be one of the most interesting and uplifting experiences of my life.

My time in Atlanta was spent with men from throughout the United States and around the world as we battled prostate cancer together. In getting to know these men, I learned their stories—all of which were fascinating, each with their own important lesson in the battle against this dreaded disease.

I wrote much of this book during my period of treatment. It is my story and a summary of stories from some of the men I spent considerable time with on our journey of hope—to be cured from prostate cancer. It outlines how we chose our treatment options. It illustrates how doctors are at odds over the best treatments available, and how many of these men made decisions about treatment after doing their own extensive research, outside the opinions of their doctors.

Our stories came together in Atlanta, Georgia, during the summer of 2000, where we had chosen Radiotherapy Clinics of Georgia for their specialized radiation treatment. Each of us believed that this clinic provided the best treatment available for us. However, this book is not intended to promote Radiotherapy Clinics of Georgia's treatment. It is up to each individual to select a treatment that is best for them.

Battling the Killer Within and Winning is intended as a valued resource to men, their wives, loved ones, or other family members who may be responsible for helping to manage their health care. The book will educate and make you aware of prostate cancer risk levels and screening guidelines. A personal "Prostate Health Management Guide" to help you understand, record, and interpret your prostate health monitoring results is included as an appendix.

For men newly diagnosed and facing prostate cancer or men on the survival journey looking for renewed hope, this book will help you conquer fear. It will assist in your understanding of various treatment options and which may be best for you.

I also hope that *Battling the Killer Within and Winning* helps you to become aware of the raging war against prostate cancer and encourages you to join in this war.

Introduction

Each day, hundreds of men in the United States are told they have prostate cancer, and immediately these men are thrust into both a psychological and physical battle with a killer. However, if these battles are approached with sound knowledge and the right strategies, beating prostate cancer is very possible.

The American Cancer Society estimates there were approximately 230,000 new prostate cancer cases diagnosed in 2004. This is the leading type of cancer among men by a margin of 2 to 1 when compared to the next leading type, which is lung cancer. Prostate cancer is also the second leading cause of cancer deaths among men, with upwards of 30,000 dying from this disease each year.

According to the American Cancer Society, "While the causes of prostate cancer are not yet completely understood, researchers have found several factors that are consistently associated with an increased risk of developing this disease. Among these are age, race, nationality, diet, and family history."

Black Americans have the highest prostate cancer incidence and mortality rates in the world. However, the disease is rare in Africa, Asia, and South America. The mortality rates for black Americans more than doubles the mortality rate for white Americans, the group with the next highest level.

Prostate cancer seems to run in some families, suggesting an inherited or genetic factor. Having a father or brother with prostate cancer doubles a man's risk of developing this disease. "The risk is even higher for men with several affected relatives, particularly if their relatives were young at the time of diagnosis," according to the American Cancer Society.

Regardless of the known risk factors, prostate cancer knows no boundaries. It strikes men around the world, young and old, of all races and economic status.

Ninety-seven percent of men diagnosed with prostate cancer survive at least five years and sixty-seven percent survive at least ten years. While these numbers may seem impressive, they don't begin to tell the complete story of the havoc that prostate cancer plays on many survivors' quality of life.

I was diagnosed with prostate cancer in April 2000 at the age of 56. While prostate cancer is often characterized as a slow-growing cancer that many men will "die with" as opposed to "die from," this is not true in my family. I know this disease as "The Killer Within."

When diagnosed, I was not interested in being just a "cancer survivor"—I sought a complete cure. I wanted all the cancer cells removed from my body and I wanted to maintain my quality of life. Men can be cured from this disease, and this was my goal.

Because of my family's experience, prostate cancer is a very personal battle for me. In addition, I have two sons and many friends who are at high risk. The Journey of Hope being traveled by the men who I came to know and write about was for them, their families and friends throughout the world. We were seeking to be cured, not just treated, and we all felt that we had to find a way to beat this killer and draw the line for generations to come.

After we were diagnosed, we all seemed to have come to a shocking realization: the medical community is very fractured relative to the best treatments available to cure prostate cancer. In fact, there are no universally accepted standards as to what actually defines a cure. These factors leave most men vulnerable, at the height of their fear, facing critical life decisions.

The PSA test (Prostate Specific Antigen) to detect prostate cancer was developed in 1984. This test gained widespread use for early detection around 1990. Since then, the prostate cancer death rate has dropped. However, the medical community's position is that this drop has not conclusively proven to be a direct result of early detection screening. As a result, most major scientific and medical organizations do not advocate mass screening or even routine screening for prostate cancer.

The American Cancer Society, The American Urological Association, and National Comprehensive Cancer Network, recommend that health care providers offer the PSA blood test and digital rectal examination (DRE) yearly to men, beginning at the age of 50 who have at least a ten-year life expectancy, and to younger men who are at high risk. On the other hand, the American College of Physicians, American Society of Internal Medicine, the U.S. Preventive Services Task Force, National Cancer Institute, Centers for Disease Control and Prevention, American Association of Family Practitioners, and the American College of Preventative Medicine, do not advocate mass or routine screenings for prostate cancer.

While it is quickly evident that the medical community is at odds simply on testing alone, I find this to be most perplexing. When diagnosed with prostate cancer, the cancer is staged based upon whether the cancer is still contained within the prostate gland, moved to surrounding tissue, spread to the lymph nodes, or metastasized to other parts of the body. If the cancer is detected early, while it is still contained within the gland, treatment options and the chance for a complete cure are much better than when the cancer has spread. These are facts supported by evidence from the top prostate cancer research centers in the United States. Then why are there still medical organizations that do not support early routine screening through PSA testing?

When men are tested and found to have prostate cancer by a urologist, in every case that I know of (unless the cancer has spread into other parts of the body), surgery is recommended by the urologist. If men visit an oncologist, the oncologist will recommend radiation. How do men decide on the best treatment?

Why is it that one of the world's most renowned urologists, (Dr. Patrick Walsh at Johns Hopkins) will not perform surgery if the PSA is elevated over a certain level and the cancer is characterized as fast growing while other urologists will?

Why does the radiation treatment center with the highest cure rate in the world (Radiotherapy Clinics of Georgia) adopt a cure-rate standard the same as that for surgery, but all other radiation treatments that have trouble meeting this standard adopt a less stringent standard for cure?

These are just a few of today's critical issues surrounding the detection, treatment, and cure of prostate cancer. How did we get here?

A review of the titles of some articles that appeared in the early 1990's reveal that prostate cancer was a disease that was kept mostly silent. Consider these titles:

"The Killer We Don't Discuss" *Newsweek*, 12/27/93
"The Prostate Predicament" *Health*, 05/06/94
"The Private Pain of Prostate Cancer" *Time*, 10/05/92

"Is Your Husband Dying of Embarrassment? The Truth About Prostate Cancer" *Family Circle*, 07/20/93.

"To Kiss a Cobra: The Prostate, Man's Worst Friend" *Lets Live*, August 1993.

"Prostate Cancer: Conspiracy of Silence" *U.S. News and World Report*, 05/11/92.

"Help for the Disease Men Fear Most" *Readers Digest*, December 1992.

Prostate cancer can be a horrible disease when it is not cured. Even if it is cured, there can be serious debilitating side effects. The most severe effects include sexual impotency and urinary incontinence. I believe the stigma associated with these side effects is the primary reason that this disease remained silently in the closet until very recently.

In May 1996, Andy Grove, Chairman and CEO of Intel Corporation, wrote a story that appeared in *Fortune* magazine entitled: "Taking on Prostate Cancer." He was one of the first well-known men to step forward and talk openly about his battle with prostate cancer. Since then, other high-profile men have made their battles public. These include former United Nations Ambassador Andrew Young, General Norman Schwarzkopf, South Africa's Bishop Desmond Tutu, Yankee baseball manager, Joe Torre, and actor/singer Harry Belafonte. Financier Michael Milken, diagnosed in 1993, has become a leading financial supporter and advocate of prostate cancer research initiatives.

However, while prostate cancer is now slowly coming out of the closet, its detection and treatment is still hampered by a fractured medical community. This seems to be a result of doctors and their organizations protecting vested interests, since no other plausible explanation appears when certain positions are strongly maintained by doctors and medical organizations in the face of contradicting facts. As a result, tens of thousands of curable men diagnosed each year are receiving treatments that will not cure their cancers and they are suffering needlessly. Also, tens of thousands of other men, not yet diagnosed with prostate cancer, will not receive a PSA test early enough to give them the best chance for an ultimate cure.

In his 1996 *Fortune* magazine article, Andy Grove made these observations: "Each medical specialty. . . surgery, cryosurgery, different branches of radiology. . . favored its own approach. I listened to the audiotape of a long interdisciplinary medical meeting called, appropriately enough, Prostate Cancer Shootout. I could sense the undercurrents of strong disagreement, couched in polite, faux, respectful terms. I had the impression that the people whose comments I heard had made the exact same comments in meetings before this one and would make them again in the future. The tenors always sang tenor; the baritones, baritone; and the basses, bass. As a patient whose life and well-being depended on a meeting of the minds, I realized I would have to do some cross-disciplinary work on my own." Andy Grove went on to point out: ". . . medical practitioners primarily tended to publish their own data; they often didn't compare their data with the data of other practitioners, even in their own field, let alone with the results of other types of treatments for the same condition. So I kept on doing cross-comparisons as best I could."

Well, I can emphatically say that Andy Grove's observations still hold true. I will also emphasize that, like Dr. Grove, all of the men who I met during my treatment did their own cross-comparisons, and they were all very sophisticated men capable of these analyses, with the time and resources to do so.

My father was not able to perform the analysis that would have led him to the best treatments available, and neither will tens of thousands of other men. As opposed to undergoing major surgery, my father chose hormonal therapy. This treatment does not provide a cure and will be chosen by other men for the same reason as my father, and in too many instances, the end result will be the same—death.

In spite of the medical community being fractured over prostate care and cancer treatment, I hold this community in very high esteem. It has made tremendous strides in developing technologies and procedures to treat and cure prostate cancer. Then where is the problem?

Men have come a long way on the prostate cancer journey. From keeping this disease closeted to now publicly stepping forward, men have made important strides. Now it is critical that we run the last mile of this journey, otherwise many of the medical gains will not be known and available to *all* of the 200,000 plus men diagnosed each year in the United States and countless others worldwide. The "last mile" has to be a period of concerted activism. Women made breast cancer awareness and treatment a priority and they have done an excellent job. We must do the same with prostate cancer and create a visible and strong prostate cancer movement. Men must become the catalyst to bring clarity to the detection and treatment of prostate cancer. The medical community has proven, over the past decade (since the widespread use of PSA testing), that it is incapable of taking us the last mile without a strong and active catalyst.

We should not be dismayed and dissuaded that our active involvement is necessary at this point in the prostate cancer battle, but excited and relieved that there are truly good and proven medical treatment options available.

Chapter I
Sweet Victory

It was a beautiful Saturday June morning, the sky was cloudless and the temperature was perfect. On days like these, my historic New England town is an ideal place to be. My wife, Juarez, had traveled to Cape Town, South Africa, to visit Tomeeka, our daughter, and I was home alone. I decided, as I often do, to have breakfast at the local West Concord Donut Shop—an unassuming place that serves a good breakfast. A young family, Rick and Karen Dee, own it and I always enjoy watching them work together, especially with their four little girls, the oldest seemingly no more than ten. They reminded me of the way my family worked together when I was growing up.

As I enjoyed my breakfast on this tranquil and peaceful day, I had no way of suspecting that this was the beginning of the most turbulent and challenging twelve months of my life.

A stranger asked to borrow my newspaper, and after I gave it to him I overheard him and Karen discussing a diet. I asked him about it. I let him know that I had been diagnosed with diabetes about eighteen months earlier, and that I was interested in understanding healthy dieting. He suddenly became eager to explain the diet he was following. He said it was good for diabetics and that I should purchase a book, *The New Diet Revolution*, by Dr. Atkins, and learn more.

I have often asked Karen about the stranger who I met by chance that Saturday morning, but she had never seen him before or since that fateful day. Today, I refer to him as my angel.

I had never been into any type of serious dieting program. I was slightly overweight and suffered from diabetes. After thinking about it, I decided to go to the local pharmacy to buy the book. Since I was home alone, I had time to kill anyway. I easily located the book and when I returned home, began to skim through the contents to see what it was all about. Dr. Atkins identified insulin as the fat-producing hormone in his book and explained controlling not only weight with his diet, but also diabetes without using medication. I had been taking two medications Glucophage and Glyburide twice daily to control my diabetes. I disliked the side effects of these drugs, in fact, I had taken myself off the Glyburide solely because of the side effects.

The Atkins book was intriguing. It put things into perspective for me relative to food, nutrition and diabetes. Never before had it been presented as convincingly as in this book. Dr. Atkins very accurately described how I felt physically, so I knew there had to be some validity to what he was saying. I completed the book that weekend and immediately began the Atkins diet.

I followed the diet very strictly, checking my blood sugar level three times each day. After only four days of this, I was able to come off my medication for diabetes! I could not believe what I had been able to accomplish with the Atkins diet plan and nutritional supplements.

Born and raised in Chapel Hill, North Carolina, my normal diet was, without question, based on the good soul foods of the South. I had to give up at least fifty percent of the foods that I had enjoyed all of my life. This included desserts, milk, fruit, fruit juices, cereal, bread (except for occasional whole grain), and other foods high in sugar and carbohydrates.

As soon as I realized I could control my diabetes without medication, I readily gave up my lifelong eating habits.

My father had suffered from diabetes since his mid-forties, was on insulin since his diagnosis, and I had painfully watched diabetes completely destroy his quality of life. I was there with him as they took off his first leg, then his second, watched him begin dialysis, and saw him struggle to maintain sight in one eye after diabetes had taken the sight from the other. I watched my mother and sister care for him as his health continued to decline over the years.

My father was always an energetic man, full of life. Even now, in this state, he was mentally the strongest man I had ever known. Not once had I heard him complain about his condition. Each time he came out of the operating room after they amputated his legs, he smiled, and somehow that smile consoled our family.

The chance to avoid the ravages of diabetes drove me to become a strong adherent to my new way of eating. Seeing my father's life change so dramatically, I was determined to make whatever sacrifices necessary.

When I stopped taking medication for diabetes, I essentially removed myself from the doctor's care. Juarez's work experience and education had been in medical technology and health administration and she meticulously managed the family's health care. She continually urged me to visit the doctor to make sure I wasn't doing anything wrong. Stubbornly, I told her that I would, once I had proven to myself that this plan was effective.

From June to September 1999, I stayed with my dieting program and lost thirty pounds. My blood sugar levels were ideal, usually between 70 to 100. I regained energy that I didn't realize could be summoned from my body. I felt, and looked, great.

I decided that it was now time to visit my doctor and get a full examination to ensure that I was well.

During the physical, my doctor noted my blood sugar level with approval, and asked if I was still properly taking my medication. I informed him that I hadn't taken any since June and that I was able to manage the diabetes with my diet. He approved, and said as long as I maintained the diet, and a normal blood sugar level, I shouldn't expect any major side effects from the diabetes.

My health had been very good throughout my life, now I had gotten my diabetes under control. This was a wonderful triumph. Knowing that I could avoid the fate that my father had suffered with diabetes, I was fully committed to my new eating habits!

From a chance meeting with a stranger over breakfast, I was driven to learn more about my body and health than I had ever known. I also now understood how important self-discipline was to a healthy lifestyle. I had lost weight, gained a renewed energy, and was feeling great. I was excited to direct this additional energy back into my business and enjoying life.

Chapter II
Signs of Prostate Cancer

One week later as I celebrated my sweet victory, I received some disturbing news about my PSA from the physical exam. It had risen to 5.8. I was not overly concerned about this news because my PSA had been steadily creeping upward over the past four to five years, and my doctor always performed a digital rectal examination (DRE) without finding a problem. However, in a note sent along with my PSA test results, my doctor advised me to come in for another PSA reading in December.

While my father's most visible physical problems were all attributable to diabetes, he was also suffering from prostate cancer. He had chosen to completely disregard prostate cancer when he was informed of his high PSA. He didn't want to wage a battle with this disease as he was struggling so much with diabetes. Consequently, I never focused on prostate cancer at the same level as diabetes, which was most visible each time I saw my father.

At this point, my father was on hormone treatment and his doctors told us that the prostate cancer was progressing. However, I still didn't have a good understanding of prostate cancer and I saw no visible signs of him struggling with it.

I went back to enjoying life without having to deal with the daily side effects of the diabetes medication, and with the peace of mind that I could avoid the ravages of diabetes. Also, as we approached the new millennium, my information technology business was very busy preparing customers for this unknown phenomena. We had to assure our clients that their computer systems would not "blow-up" on January 1, 2000. Not once had I focused on the probability that I had a prostate problem.

We spent Thanksgiving of 1999 at our home in Chapel Hill, North Carolina, to be with my parents and my sister and her family. When I saw my father, I was struck by how much his health had declined since I had last seen him two months earlier. My father and I had always been very close. He was a man I had great admiration for, and had been the driving force in shaping my life along with my mother. When I was married he was my best man, and my two sons, Christopher and Trevor, and daughter, Tomeeka, adored him. To see him struggling was painful for me. Even now, his strength was unbelievable. He dressed himself and took care of his personal needs each day as he left home for the dialysis clinic.

After I returned to Massachusetts following Thanksgiving, I had a difficult time psychologically, dealing with my father's health issues. As his condition worsened, I returned to Chapel Hill in little more than a week to be with him again. While he was hospitalized I spent a lot of time with him in the hospital and had a chance to talk extensively with his doctors. It was clear that his days on this earth were drawing to a close. My mother, my sister, Gerri, and Juarez and I had to discuss the fate of my father, as a family group. We each knew that time was drawing near but, privately, each of us held out hope that a miracle would be sent down from heaven and he would regain his strength and be with us a while longer. We all had gone through so much together and witnessed so many miracles in our lives, we were praying for just one more.

We dreaded the thought of life without the man who had been part of the very foundation of our lives, and through his personality, always brought joy and laughter to our family. After a week, dad was released from the hospital and returned home. We wanted desperately to believe it was due to him regaining strength, but the doctors let us know that there was simply nothing else that could be done for him.

On Christmas Eve, prostate cancer took my father's life. My entire family came to Chapel Hill for the funeral, where we remained until after the New Year. December had been so trying and hectic that I never once remembered my doctor's note to have my PSA tested as a follow-up to the September exam.

At the dawn of the new millennium, just a couple of weeks following my father's funeral, my worst nightmare began to play out as my mother was hospitalized for a recurrence of her heart problem. I was back in North Carolina to be with her. All during my father's last days, I was worried sick about the impact this strain could have on my mother's health. She suffered from congestive heart failure and had a combination pacemaker and defibrillator permanently implanted some years earlier. Seeing her in the same hospital, where I had just spent time with my father a month earlier, was a chilling experience. While my customer's computer systems worked fine during the millennium crossover, it seemed that our close-knit family was blowing up and I was helpless to do anything about it.

Through prayer and God's blessings, my mother recovered from her problems and was released from the hospital. The family was thankful and breathed a sigh of relief, we could move on without the worries of my mother's health and reflect on the memories of all the good times we had with my father, realizing that his spirit remained a part of us all and that he would forever be present.

In late March, I received a note from my doctor reminding me that I had not been back for my PSA test. How could I have overlooked this? I scheduled the test immediately. The results showed that my PSA had risen to 6.4. Also, my doctor noted on the results something about the "percent free PSA" count being too low at 7%. He wanted me to see a urologist and have a prostate biopsy. Suddenly, this prostate situation had my attention for the very first time.

On Monday, April 10, I visited the urologist for my biopsy. I had heard horror stories about this procedure. The urologist and a technician used an ultrasonic guided probe that was inserted in the rectum. This probe had needles that were shot out of it to obtain tissue samples from the prostate gland. While this was not a pleasant procedure by any means, it was not the horrific experience that I had heard about. As the urologist stared at the ultrasound scan, he told me an irregularity had been detected on one side of the prostate. My prostate problem had now gotten my full attention.

As I lay in the recovery room after the biopsy, I began to realize that I knew absolutely nothing about the prostate, what function it performed, and what types of problems I would have, should my biopsy be positive. With my family's history, I wondered how I could be so ignorant about the prostate. But even as I lay there, I could not imagine the biopsy result would show cancer. I had never had a pain or any other type of prostate problem. My doctor had always given me a digital rectal exam during regular physicals and found nothing, and I certainly was not sick.

Two days after my biopsy, I was scheduled to go to Chapel Hill to visit with my mother. The urologist indicated that he would have the results while I was in Chapel Hill. I decided not to mention a word of this to my mother, as she was still trying to recover after losing my father to prostate cancer and from her own illness.

While I was in Chapel Hill, my mother, Gerri, and I scheduled time to look at tombstones for my father's gravesite. After speaking to a tombstone maker, we decided to visit a few cemeteries to view how the tombstones that we liked looked in an actual setting. This was my very first experience shopping for a tombstone, and it was a strange feeling as I missed my father so very much.

As we toured these cemeteries, we visited the gravesites of my father and both my grandfathers. We first visited Hamlet's Chapel, the resting place of my mother's father, Thomas Wesley Gattis, a prostate cancer victim. After a while we journeyed to my home church, Terrell's Creek Baptist. Their resting places—my father, Osmond Thomas Farrington, Jr., and his father, Osmond Thomas Farrington, Sr., also a prostate cancer victim—are located very close to each other. As I walked between their graves I could not help but reflect on these two men and what they had meant to my life. I always knew I was blessed because they had taught me so much about life, particularly how to be a man. They both had been role models and mentors. My father was gregarious, always the life of the party with a keen mind and incredible wit. While my grandfather was a quiet man, deeply religious and strongly committed to our church.

In addition to being the only son, I was also the oldest grandson and my relationships with these two men were near perfect. Regardless of where I was or what challenge I had to overcome in my life, it was their teachings and examples that I always felt comfortable relying on. They were two strong, fiercely independent, caring, and gentle men, and I loved them so, but prostate cancer took them both. As I continued to move back and forth between their resting places, I could feel their spirits as I recalled all the good times we shared, but I also began to really understand that prostate cancer is a vicious killer, and within my family it is a serial killer. Like an invisible alien, prostate cancer had invaded the bodies of the men in my family and fearlessly moved from generation to generation. I was next in line. Standing in the cemetery, this sobering realization heightened my anxiety over the biopsy results, but it also angered me; this killer was attacking my family with such abandon.

When we returned from the cemeteries, I hurriedly called my office and learned that my urologist had not called with the biopsy results. I figured that no news was good news. With no bad news, I did my best to enjoy a peaceful weekend with my family.

Chapter III
Facing Prostate Cancer

On Tuesday morning, April 18, 2000, Sharon, my longtime administrative assistant came to my office to let me know that my urologist was on the telephone. At last the call that will convey the message that everything was fine, I thought. When I got on the phone my doctor's words, as best as I can remember, went something like this: "The biopsy results came back positive. You have prostate cancer—but, don't panic. . . ." As I panicked, my first response was to ask why he had not contacted me with the results earlier. I don't remember his answer. I sat at my desk, stunned, shocked, and in total disbelief. . . . I have cancer! How can this be? Fear immediately set in.

I sat alone at my desk for what seemed like an eternity, not ready to accept what I had heard. Juarez realized I had gotten the news and rushed in to my office and closed the door to shield my shock from the staff. She then summoned Trevor and Tomeeka, both of whom were in the office. After we all settled down a bit and I was able to stand, we went out of the office to spend some time talking. Not only was this a major blow for me, but also for my family as we sat in the restaurant trying to grasp what this all meant. Juarez is a strong person and she was not about to let our family gathering turn into a gloom and doom session, even though she was as much at a loss for explanations as we all were. Trevor had been at my side in our business for a number of years and understood my various moods and how to deal with them. He now faced one he had not witnessed before, but he tried to assure me that this would somehow work itself out and I would be fine. Tomeeka, our youngest child, was in the midst of planning her college graduation. Another family health crisis was not what she was hoping for, but like her mother, she stayed strong and helped allay my visible state of shock at hearing the news. After we were together for quite some time, my shock gave way to the reality that I had to face prostate cancer, and I had no idea what that meant, other than I knew I was facing a killer. This alien had moved into my body and I now had the killer within.

Christopher, our oldest, was living in New York City. Juarez called him with the news and I spoke with him for a while. Quiet and reserved by nature, Chris didn't let this news cause him to panic. He added his words of support and encouragement. With the immediate family informed, the decision was to make no further announcements until we were able to understand the complete prognosis. I didn't want to waste any time so I spent the remainder of the day and most of the evening on the Internet searching for an understanding of prostate cancer before my appointment with the urologist the next day.

As I began my learning process, I felt totally amazed at my lack of awareness of the prostate and complete ignorance of prostate cancer considering my family history. But, I had never fully connected my family's history to the fact that I was at risk for prostate cancer, until just a few days earlier.

My research began at a very basic level: What is the prostate and what does it do?

I discovered that the prostate gland is about the size of an egg. It is located in my pelvis between my bladder (at the top) and my rectum (at the bottom). The prostate consists of millions of cells, which are surrounded by a thin covering called the capsule, much like the shell of an egg. The top of the prostate next to the bladder, is called the base. The bottom of this gland is called the apex. Lying against the prostate on each side, near the apex, are sex nerves. Running through the middle of the prostate is the urethra, the tube that goes from the bladder out through the penis for urination. The sex nerves take part in causing an erection of the penis, and the prostate produces semen, the material ejaculated during sexual orgasm. Treatments that remove or damage the sex nerves can cause erectile dysfunction, also known as impotence.

What news! I thought as I learned more about the prostate. This is an important organ that I never really knew anything about. I continued my research to gain a better understanding of what prostate cancer is and how it is treated.

It seemed that the cause of prostate cancer is not fully understood, but it begins when one or more normal cells inside the prostate transform into cancer cells. Prostate cancer then enters the first of three phases of growth.

Phase 1: Growth inside the prostate contained by the capsule. Prostate cancer cells multiply and grow inside the prostate with growth contained by the capsule.

Phase 2: Penetration of the capsule and growth into the surrounding normal organs. In this phase, cancer cells penetrate through the prostate capsule and extend into surrounding normal organs including the rectum, sex nerves, bladder, and into the muscles that control urination. These "microscopic capsule penetration" cancer cells continue to multiply.

Phase 3: Spread, called metastasis, by lymph and blood vessels to other parts of the body. In the third and final phase of prostate cancer, microscopic capsule penetration cancer cells, or cancer cells inside the prostate, invade lymph nodes or blood vessels. Using lymph nodes and blood vessels as a highway, prostate cancer cells spread throughout the body. Initially, metastasis usually go to lymph nodes and bones, later affecting the lungs, liver and other parts of the body.

What I also learned from my Internet research was that prostate cancer could be cured if it was detected and eradicated during phase 1. If it was allowed to spread and metastasize, it was incurable. On the Internet, I read accounts of men and their horrific battles—death came steadily marching through all treatments that were thrown against it when this cancer was allowed to spread. This was a frightening first glimpse of prostate cancer—my disease. While I found little time for sleep, I found plenty of time to pray and ask God for strength and His blessing.

As I went to meet with my urologist the following morning, I was more knowledgeable about prostate cancer, and much more afraid of what I might learn from his analysis of my situation. As Juarez and I sat in the doctor's office waiting to be seen, I was still in a state of shock and disbelief that I had cancer. How could I sit calmly and wait to have this discussion, I thought.

My urologist patiently began to discuss my test results. First, he let me know that my prostate was not really enlarged, it was just slightly above the normal size. Then he told me that of the six biopsy tissue samples that had been taken, cancer was found in three of them. Cancer appeared at both the left and right apex and the right mid of the gland. The cancer grade was deemed to be a Gleason Grade 7. I didn't know, at this point, the significance of this data, but I was about to learn.

In a calming manner that I shall never forget, my urologist began to talk about treatment options. He pointed out that surgery was the "gold standard" treatment recommended by most urologists. He cited radiation treatment as an option. As I was still grappling with the meaning of this discussion, he dropped a bombshell—my urologist began to talk about a nerve-sparing surgery technique that he and others had used to try and keep the sex nerves intact. For my case, however, he could not use this procedure, and I would come out of surgery impotent! With cancer located on both sides of the apex, where the sex nerves are located, nerve-sparing surgery was not possible.

As we sat, shocked and in disbelief yet again, my urologist began to talk about penile implants, shots and other methods of getting an erection. Juarez and I stared at each other. She put her hand gently on my back, trying to provide some reassurance. My God, I thought, when is this going to end? First cancer, now impotence. It was just the beginning.

A Gleason Grade 7 is classified as an aggressive or moderately aggressive cancer. My urologist wanted me to undergo a series of tests before we decided on any treatment. These tests were to determine whether cancer had spread beyond the prostate to other parts of the body. My mind immediately flashed back to what I had seen on the Internet the night before, accounts of the suffering and deaths of men who had not caught this disease before it spread. Was this to be my plight?

As Juarez and I stumbled out of the urologist's office, I realized that we had been totally unprepared for what had just taken place. While Juarez was still trying to console me, I didn't know how I was supposed to respond to hearing that I was soon to be impotent, assuming I had a chance to be cured. This was about as bad as it could get, I thought.

My urologist had scheduled the appointments for the necessary tests. The problem was that they were scheduled a week from this day. This was going to be a very tough week—the anticipation, the unknown, and the fear. I would have to balance all of these factors as I awaited word of my fate. My doctor suggested that I try to stay away from the Internet for a while. He thought it would only serve to heighten my anxiety, and much of what I would find would be put there by non-doctors, he claimed.

I returned home and immediately dialed onto the Internet to try and understand the upcoming tests and what to expect. I gained enough knowledge to take my fear and anxiety to a higher level. I learned some of the symptoms of cancer metastasis. This turned out to be the longest week of my life, as it seemed that I experienced each and every symptom I had read about.

At this time, I also told Sharon and others in my office about my condition and my plans for treatment. Surely, Sharon suspected something with the various doctor and lab visits, but she was not expecting me to announce that I had cancer. She and I had been together for thirteen years and I considered her family. She immediately began to look for ways to support and help me face this new challenge.

While I considered myself a strong person, this experience took its toll on me. It was extremely tough sleeping nights as I awaited the tests. Also, I had eventually taken my doctor's advice and stopped trying to learn anything else about prostate cancer. I was going to trust in his care. I only wished the day of testing would hurry up and arrive.

When the day came for my testing, April 24, 2000, I experienced a sense of relief, along with fear and anxiety. At last I would know whether the cancer had spread; but what if it had? Juarez and I went to the hospital laboratory for these tests. She had such a calming presence as I waited impatiently. I had a bone scan and a CAT scan performed.

Before I left the hospital, I learned that the bone scan was negative, but I had to await the CAT scan results. I was feeling much better knowing the results of the bone scan. The next day I learned that the CAT scan was also negative. What a relief!   At least I have a chance of battling this killer within, I thought. At last we had stopped the downward spiral. With the good news, our immediate family came together to celebrate a positive step forward. Understanding that we were still faced with a monumental battle, I was feeling good for the first time in quite a while.

I met with my urologist again to talk about finalizing a treatment plan. When we met this time, I was in a much better frame of mind. It seemed that we had caught this cancer early enough to cure it. In our discussions, we resumed talks about surgery and radiation treatments. My urologist would perform the surgery that, he felt, could remove all the cancer. I would, he advised again, be impotent from this procedure. Believing that surgery would cure me of cancer and concluding that if I were not cured, then the issue of sexual potency was irrelevant, I decided to have surgery. Searching for a second opinion, I went to another urologist with all of my test results. He confirmed what my original urologist had said. Based on all of this data and information, I was now ready to schedule surgery.

Tomeeka was graduating from Boston College on May 23rd. Juarez and I decided on surgery for May 25th, because I didn't want to be incapacitated on my daughter's big day, and this would present an opportunity to break the news to my mother during her visit for graduation.

Over the next month, I tried to get things in place in anticipation of being away from my business during surgery and recovery. Also, for three consecutive weeks leading up to surgery, I went to the blood bank to have blood drawn in preparation. Surgery was scheduled at Emerson Hospital in my town of Concord. My bed was allocated. Everything was set.

I chose a radical prostatectomy for treatment. In this operation, the entire prostate gland, plus some surrounding tissue, is removed. A radical prostatectomy is used most often if the cancer is "thought" not to have spread outside the gland (Phase 1). There are two main types of radical prostatectomy (a) radical retropubic prostatectomy, and (b) radical perineal prostatectomy. My surgery was to be the retropubic operation where an incision is made in the abdomen to remove the prostate gland. The nerve-sparing procedure is a modification of this operation. If it appears that the cancer has not spread to these nerves, the surgeon will not remove them. Leaving them intact lowers, but does not eliminate, the risk of not being able to have an erection (impotence).

This surgery was expected to keep me in the hospital for five days, and convalescing at home for up to six weeks. I would be fitted with a catheter for up to three weeks. This is a major surgery and the risks associated with a radical prostatectomy are similar to those of any major surgery. These include the potential for heart attack, stroke, blood clots in the legs that may travel to the lungs, and infection at the incision site. In rare cases, death can occur as a result of this operation.

The main side effects of radical prostatectomy are incontinence and impotence. During the radical prostatectomy procedure, the urethra is severed from the bladder to remove the prostate gland then it is surgically reconnected. However, in some cases the muscles that control urine flow are damaged. This creates an inability to completely control the urine flow (incontinence). Mild stress incontinence, which is passing a small amount of urine when coughing, laughing, sneezing, or exercising, may persist permanently after surgery in up to 35% of men. About 10% of patients have more serious stress, which may be permanent. Approximately 2% of men report complete loss of bladder control and another 7% have frequent leakage of urine. About 20% of men use absorbent pads because of incontinence.

Studies have found that if surgery does not remove the nerves on either side of the prostate, the impotence rate is as low as 25% to 30% for men under the age of 60. Other studies have reported higher rates of impotence in similar patients. Impotence occurs in 70% to 80% of men over the age of 70. If potency remains after surgery, orgasm should continue to be pleasurable, but there is no ejaculation of semen. The orgasm is dry.

I approached surgery understanding the risks, and the fact that I would become impotent. While this was not a comforting thought, I chose this treatment because I knew that if I was not cured of prostate cancer, it would some day kill me, as it had my father and grandfathers. I fully expected prostate cancer to be completely removed from my body with the radical surgery.

My urologist had discussed various methods of achieving an erection after surgery. One approach is a penile implant. I spoke to a friend who had this surgery performed five years earlier and he was doing fine with no signs of cancer recurrence. He had a penile implant and told me that he now has the best sex of his life. I had never used Viagra and now it didn't quite look like I would have that need, but after this conversation with my friend, I thought that maybe a penile implant was the best way to achieve a higher level of sexuality. I certainly hoped so. I was anxious to be cured of prostate cancer and move on with as much of my life left intact as possible. Sex was an important part.

Chapter IV
Graduation Weekend

As the weekend for Tomeeka's graduation and my surgery date rapidly approached, I was confident that I had somehow prepared myself for prostate cancer treatments. I still had not spoken with my mother or sister about my condition. I had decided that I needed to be with my mother when I gave her the news. I asked her to come to Concord early, before the graduation festivities got underway, though, I had not told her why. I was so concerned about her health, and how she was going to take the news. She scheduled her trip to arrive in Boston on Thursday, May 18th, and she agreed to stay for a week or two following the graduation.

This was going to be a very busy four days for our family. We were expecting six houseguests, family and friends, who would begin arriving on Friday, May 19th. Juarez was president of her Links chapter that was hosting an event on Saturday evening featuring nationally acclaimed entertainer, Jennifer Holliday, and she was very busy helping put this event together. We were having a graduation party for Tomeeka at our home on Sunday, and Monday was graduation day. After all of the festivities, there was just a one-day break (Tuesday), before I was to enter the hospital for surgery. All of this activity helped keep my mind off my condition.

My urologist's office was located very close to my home, so I went by his facility each day as I traveled to and from my office. On Monday, prior to graduation weekend, I decided to stop by his office to see if he had time to chat about the upcoming surgery. He wasn't available, but his office administrator insisted that she would make sure he telephoned me sometime during the week, but as the week progressed, I didn't hear from him. Anyway, I didn't think too much of it; I was all set for surgery, and everything was in place.

On Wednesday, Trevor went to the airport and picked up my mother. She was excited about Tomeeka's graduation and anxiously waiting for me to tell her why I wanted her to come early and stay longer. She was expecting me to unveil some exciting plans. This was very difficult. After she was settled in and had a chance to relax, I decided to tell her. I could not put it off any longer. I sat down next to her, held her hands and said, I have some bad news and some good news. She looked alarmed. I continued, the bad news is that I have prostate cancer, and quickly said, the good news is that we have caught it early enough to cure it. My mother began to cry, "no ... no ... no ...." I spent some time comforting her while maintaining my composure, which was tough, but I had to stay positive.

I talked to my mother about what I had gone through, the urologist's assessments and the fact that on the following Wednesday, all of the prostate cancer would be removed from my body through surgery, and I would be fine. I was not sure that she concurred with what I was saying, but after a while she calmed down and seemed to be doing somewhat better, which was my primary concern at this stage.

Later that evening, my mother called home to talk with Gerri, my only sibling, and to inform her about my prostate cancer. According to my mother, Gerri took it very hard. Gerri had moved in with my parents as my father's health continued to decline, and she had been there with my mother to interface with the doctors. Over a period of time, she developed a total disdain for doctors. While she relied upon their care for our father, she questioned their every diagnosis and treatment.

Whenever my father's doctors would make a diagnosis, she, or her son, Kurtis, or daughter, Nicole, would immediately go to the Internet to understand, and question, the doctor's every move.

My father and I often talked about her confrontations with his doctors because he was concerned that the doctors would possibly take their anger out on him. I repeatedly told Gerri that the doctors knew medicine and what was best, and she could not expect to go to the Internet to get information, and then question the doctor's directions. My sister was always strong-willed and no amount of convincing was about to change her perspective on doctors. In her mind, she had seen them make too many mistakes to be trusted.

Gerri was also flying into Boston on Saturday for the graduation. I had planned to talk with her then. However, she called me back and immediately said she felt prostate surgery was the wrong treatment. She told me that while our father was being treated for prostate cancer, she had read information on a natural healing approach that had worked for men. I listened and politely told her that I would, indeed, look into it. True to my word, I went to the Internet and located the Web page of the leader of this natural healing approach. I am an engineer by training, and I always look for the hard data, facts and proof. My sister is a sociologist by training, and she, most times, will take an opposite approach to solving a problem. After studying the information on the natural healing approach, I could not find enough hard data for it to hold my serious attention, but I did find another Web page advocating alternative treatment. The next day, I purchased a book by the proponent of this approach, which included herbal remedies, fasting and dietary changes. The book was a real eye opener. However, I still had no intentions of abandoning my surgical treatment for a natural healing approach that only had one subject, the author, that it referenced to prove its merits.

On Friday afternoon, after not hearing from my urologist since stopping by his office on Monday, I finally got him on the telephone. I told him that I had no questions, but simply wanted to touch base with him before going into surgery the following Wednesday. We chatted briefly, and I told him how pleased I was that we caught this cancer early enough to be able to cut it all out and be done with it. Shockingly, he responded by saying that we really would not know if we got it all until after surgery. I asked him to explain, since the tests that I had taken showed no spread of cancer. What was the issue? He said that after the prostate gland is removed, a pathologist would examine tissue under a microscope to determine if there had been any microscopic cancer cell penetration outside the gland. He further explained that the tests that I had taken would not reveal such "microscopic capsule penetration." Are you telling me that I can have surgery and still have prostate cancer?" His response was, "Yes, but. . . ." My mind blocked out his voice. I didn't hear another word.

As I sat at home in my office, with my mother watching television in the family room, tears began to roll down my face. In all that I had gone through, this was the first and only time I cried. This news seemed to have jolted my entire body like an electrical shock.

I was struggling to absorb what I had just heard. My urologist told me that after surgery, where I would certainly be impotent, maybe incontinent, or even worse, I could still end up with prostate cancer in my body. Maybe he had briefly discussed this with me before, but I certainly didn't recall it and I didn't know how I could have missed it. I found this news to be more devastating than when he originally told me I had cancer. After a while, I did two things. First, I prayed again. I hoped God was not getting tired of hearing from me, because I had been on the prayer line quite frequently over the past few weeks. Secondly, I made a pact with myself that I was going to take control of this prostate problem and understand every single thing that I possibly could about this cancer and its treatment. Maybe my sister had been correct all along in her response to doctors, that their diagnoses were more akin to a sociological solution than an engineering final answer and, open for debate.

It was Friday afternoon and I was scheduled to go into surgery the following Wednesday morning, my time was very short.

My home had become a very busy place as guests arrived and preparations for the next three days activities were well underway. In fact, I was supposed to help out, and I tried to fake it as best I could. However, after everyone settled in, I spent the entire night on my computer.

My Internet research was beginning to pay off. On microscopic capsule penetration I found the results of a study performed at Johns Hopkins University by Dr. Partin. Dr. Partin had analyzed the results of pathologists' post-surgical data that showed actual microscopic capsule penetration based on patients' pre-treatment PSA levels. He used his research to develop a widely accepted set of data called the "Partin Table." This table is used within the medical field as a guide to determine the probability of microscopic capsule penetration for those diagnosed with prostate cancer

Partin Table*

PSA Group	% with Microscopic Capsule Penetration
0.0 – 4.0 ng/ml	25%
4.1 – 10.0 ng/ml	50%
10.1 – 20.0 ng/ml	75%
20.1 ng/ml or more	Almost All

*See Appendix 17 for updated data.

My PSA was 6.4. Using the Partin Table, there was a 50% probability that cancer cells had spread beyond my prostate gland. If microscopic cancer cells are left behind after surgery, they will grow, and my post-treatment PSA will rise, clearly signaling cancer recurrence.

My reaction was that 50% odds are horrible odds when considering life and death. These are the same odds as a coin flip, and I would never knowingly use a coin flip to determine whether I live or die. However, my interpretation of the Partin Table clearly showed that it was precisely what I would be doing with prostate surgery. This was the most profound realization that came out of my Friday night of research. As I finally slipped into bed around 5 a.m., still wide awake, I contemplated my next move.

Saturday was much more hectic. Things were moving fast and furious, but I was in slow motion. Everyone was getting ready for the Jennifer Holliday event. Since Juarez was part of the program, she was busy making sure that it was going to be successful. I told everyone to make themselves at home, and I got back on the Internet. I don't like these odds, I kept saying to myself, but what options did I have? I had not really had any substantive discussions with my urologist on other treatments. Are there any treatments that may be better than surgery, I wondered. My urologist had only told me that I would have one good shot of curing prostate cancer. He had described surgery as the gold standard. Did this mean that there are no better options? I continued to question myself.

When I got on the Internet this time, I decided to look up radiation treatments. My urologist had mentioned radiation, but hadn't discussed it any further with me. What I found were many different types: external beam, Brachytherapy (seed implants and high-dose rate). I studied all of these to the extent that I could, but I was becoming more confused than enlightened. How would these treatments handle my odds? It was difficult to determine. As I scrolled through the many radiation treatments and treatment facilities, I kept coming across a link to Radiotherapy Clinics of Georgia. I was in Massachusetts. What medical advancement could they possibly have in Georgia that wasn't here in Massachusetts? I continually bypassed this link.

I found and read Andy Grove's *Fortune* article, and it was fascinating. He chose a radiation treatment called high dose rate or HDR. Now, I was simply flying through information on a cursory basis to see if anything could help me with my 50% odds problem. I tried to visit Dr. Grove's treatment facility online, but didn't gain enough information to help me. As Saturday wore on, I finally decided to go to the Radiotherapy Clinics of Georgia link.

The information that I found on their Web site was revealing. Most importantly, they dealt with my "microscopic capsule penetration" problem. From first glance, it seemed that their treatment philosophy was aimed specifically at what I considered to be *my* problem.

While my knowledge at that point was very limited, it seemed that RCOG, as they refer to themselves, combined two forms of radiation treatment into a single treatment. According to the information on their Web site, this is done to kill all the cancer cells within the gland, and the microscopic capsule penetration cells that may have escaped in the surrounding areas. Maybe there was a better approach to treating my cancer than surgery. Maybe my prayers would be answered. God knows, I was very uncomfortable with coin flip odds on microscopic capsule penetration.

I wished for someone, anyone, I could talk to about my dilemma and concerns. At this point, with just a few days before I was to have surgery, it seemed that I was really on my own. While I was not unaccustomed to making decisions, I had never before been faced with one in terms of life or death.

The more I learned, the more I was beginning to question surgery as the right treatment for me. I still wasn't sure what might be the best option. While RCOG looked intriguing, I would clearly have to do more work understanding and analyzing their treatment. Maybe the Andy Grove treatment approach was best. I really didn't know. What I did know was that my research was over for the evening. Juarez was back, and it was time to go to her Links event. While I briefly considered not attending, I decided this would cause more distractions than I could deal with.

I knew just about everyone in attendance, and I hoped they could not sense that I wasn't really there that evening. Throughout the evening my mind was completely consumed with my research. As I watched Jennifer Holliday perform, my mind raced from one set of data to another, and I tried to make some sense of what I had learned in just two days.

My mother, sister, sister-in-law, and friends staying at our home for graduation all attended the Jennifer

Holliday event. They enjoyed it, and we stayed until everyone left. This eliminated any thoughts I had of doing more research when I returned home.

Back at home, going over what I had learned, I became a little overwhelmed. I thought medical science was a science. As an engineer, I was taught to first establish the facts as a basis for solving a problem. The more information I gathered on prostate cancer the less I became sure what facts were being held constant. RCOG talked about cure rates in their information. It was difficult to find this level of detail anywhere else. My urologist never talked about his cure rate. This is what I became most interested in knowing. I wanted a treatment with as close to a 100% cure rate as possible and hard data to back it up.

My urologist had strongly emphasized that in treating prostate cancer there really was just one good shot at beating it. This was one of the reasons I had chosen surgery. During my research, I had been able to understand the frightening progression of this disease if it were not cured. Prostate cancer is fed by testosterone, and when it isn't cured, the typical progression follows this course:

Phase 1: Treatment. Assume surgery.

Phase 2: It is determined that cancer cells were left behind, i.e., the surgery failed.

Phase 3: External beam radiation. This is an attempt to kill cancer cells that were left behind in the prostate gland area. This may or may not complete a cure.

Phase 4: Hormone treatment. Hormone treatment is a chemical castration to reduce testosterone levels and slow the growth of cancer cells.

Phase 5: The body becomes hormone resistant and cancer cells begin an aggressive growth pattern.

Phase 6: Orchiectomy. This is a surgical castration procedure to remove the testes and eliminate the source of testosterone.

Phase 7: The adrenaline glands begin to produce testosterone and again, cancer cells grow.

Phase 8: The killer wins after a battle where other treatments, including chemotherapy were used.

Battling the killer within is a long and tough journey of hope if you are not cured initially, and this journey can take many agonizing years. All throughout this journey, the patient is considered a prostate cancer survivor as long as he is alive. I certainly didn't want to have to survive this way if I could avoid it!

Tomeeka's graduation party was scheduled for Sunday. She had been a wonderful student at Boston College, and I wished I could really enjoy the weekend with her. Christopher was now home from New York. All of our immediate family was in town for the celebration. My time on the Internet ended as we prepared for the party.

We all took the trip to Boston College for graduation ceremonies on Monday. We were in the stands together as Tomeeka marched in. What a joyous time! Juarez and I were very proud parents. Now all three of our children had finished college. Christopher had his master's degree, Trevor worked with us in the business, and Tomeeka was going on to graduate school at American University in Washington, DC, in the fall to study broadcast journalism.

On this day of celebration, I sat in the stands facing one of the biggest decisions of my life. My stomach was in knots. What should I do? Was I willing to face this long journey with just flip of the coin odds? As the graduation ceremonies continued, I began to realize that this was also my graduation weekend. Tomeeka had four years to study and gain knowledge that would serve her through a lifetime and this day was the finality of that educational process. I had four days to get a prostate cancer education and on this day I had to use my knowledge to make a decision that could very well determine the rest of my life. A mandatory graduation.

Juarez and I had driven separate cars to the graduation ceremonies to transport family and friends. I returned home before she did and when I arrived, I picked up the phone and called my urologist. He was not available but I left a message with his assistant that I was canceling my surgery for Wednesday. I had made my decision. I concluded that I could not live with the 50% chance that cancer cells had penetrated the capsule and would be left behind. Shortly after, I received a return call, and a meeting was scheduled with my urologist first thing the next morning.

When Juarez and the rest of the family arrived, I told them what I had done. They were shocked. Because of the hectic pace of the weekend, I had not had a chance to talk with them in detail about my thoughts and the research I had done. I realized the impact that this unexpected announcement could have on my family. They had struggled with my condition and came to grips with the reality that it was necessary for me to undergo a major surgery and had been very supportive. Now, with no warning, I had made a "U-turn." Christopher, designated to lead a family discussion, took me into another room with Juarez, Trevor, and Tomeeka. They expressed serious concern about my decision. I sincerely apologized to them for not being able to keep them abreast of my research. Finally, they flat out asked me if I knew what I was doing. I quickly responded that I absolutely didn't know what I was doing! This was my biggest problem. I explained I had to know what I was doing before I could proceed with any type of treatment. They were still not assured that I was doing the right thing. But, I didn't have any answers, I only had questions that had to be answered before I could move forward with any type of treatment. Realizing that I could not assure them, finally I told them this was the only life that I had and I had to find the best way to keep it. I promised to keep them well informed and involved in my future decisions.

The following day I visited my urologist. He seemed shocked that I had cancelled surgery that was scheduled for the very next day. I outlined the reasons for my decision and told him it was final for now, but I would leave surgery open as an option in the future. He was understanding, and concurred that I shouldn't have surgery if I wasn't fully prepared. He advised me that I probably had this cancer for some time now and taking a few more weeks would not make a difference. I asked for his help in making appointments with a radiation treatment center and a cryosurgery center. He said he would be happy to accommodate my requests.

As I walked to my car, it dawned on me that I was no longer under a doctor's care. I was all alone facing perhaps the biggest crisis of my life. The thought shook me for a moment, but what were my options? I had made my decision, now I had to follow through with it—doctor's care, or not.

When I reached my car in the parking lot, I stared back at the medical complex in bewilderment. It was filled with doctors and medical professionals, but there was no "prostate care" professional. Yes, there were urologists, oncologists, and others who treated prostate cancer, but there was no one who I could go to for impartial consultation on this disease. Why should I sit here alone with cancer facing the monumental task of researching and analyzing various treatment options that offer me the best chance for a cure? I wondered how many of the nearly 200,000 plus men diagnosed with prostate cancer each year were faced with this same dilemma while simultaneously suffering the emotional and psychological pains of dealing with cancer. How many simply succumbed to the recommendation of surgery that surely came from most urologists—after all, they were surgeons, and surgery was the "gold standard" for prostate cancer treatment? How many urologists would even advise their patients of the microscopic capsule penetration probability factor based on their PSA reading? My urologist, while advising me of microscopic capsule penetration, never once mentioned the microscopic penetration probability factor. I wondered why I was forced to leave this medical complex with only my individual research and analytical skills to rely on.

As I continued to sit in my car, reluctant to leave this perceived lifeline of medical support, I again called on God, through prayer for guidance and support. I knew that with His blessings, I would have the strength to face the task of finding the right treatment for a cure. In all of my life's pursuits, I had called on God's power. I joined the church when I was seven years old and have always been an active worshiper. I was selected as a trustee in my original home church, Terrell's Creek Baptist, in the countryside of Chapel Hill, when I was a teenager. I remember helping to build our new church, leaving college one day to go with the other trustees to select the brick that we would use for the new building. In the Boston area, I have been a member of St. John's Baptist Church in Woburn for more than thirty years. After I first joined this church, we went through a complete renaissance. I led the planning efforts to map a new direction for the church. After some years of success, we also underwent a major building renovation. So, as I sat here facing the biggest crisis in my life, I was very comfortable calling on God for I knew God, and I had experienced His blessings throughout my life.

My mind took me back to the most recent blessing that had literally put me here at this time. Since I met that stranger at the West Concord Donut Shop almost a year earlier, my blood sugar levels remained normal and I had not needed any diabetes medication since the weekend I first met him. I had often gone back to the donut shop to ask if they had seen him again, but they hadn't. They also pointed out that they never saw him before that day. Truly, these were blessings! The examination I had taken for my blood sugar level, three months after meeting this stranger, was what detected the prostate problem. Had I not met this man I wondered would I even know, today, that I had prostate cancer? I felt that I had been touched by an angel!

Reflecting on these blessings gave me the faith that would allow me to work through my anxieties and fears and find the right treatment to cure me. I left the parking lot and I realized I was not alone, I was on a mission and I would succeed with God's help.

Chapter V
Searching for a New Battle Plan

My thoughts and activities became almost totally consumed with finding a treatment that would offer me the best chance for a complete cure. I knew nothing about the prostate or prostate cancer, and not having any medical training, my approach would have to be completely analytical. I felt that my research had given me a basis to begin this process; however, I was still shocked that this level of analysis was necessary to find the best treatment for my condition.

I decided to outline what I knew and assumed to be fact regarding my condition:

1. If prostate cancer cells had spread outside the gland and the immediate area and moved to other parts of my body, then my cancer was incurable and no treatment would offer me what I wanted. My battle plan would undertake a completely different focus. I was assuming that the tests I took showing no spread were accurate.

2. The Partin Table indicated that there was a 50% chance of microscopic cancer cell penetration outside the capsule. I had to assume that this penetration was a certainty and focus on treatments that specifically addressed this condition.

I had identified two such treatments: Radiotherapy Clinics of Georgia, (RCOG) and the treatment that Intel President, Andy Grove, chose, called the High Dose Rate (HDR) or "smart bomb".

I became intrigued by what I was able to gather over the Internet about RCOG's treatment. They provided a lot of data and information on their Web site that was educational and I decided to use this information as a template in understanding and comparing other treatments.

RCOG offered cure-rate data for both five- and ten-year periods after treatment. This data, like the Partin Table, was broken down by pre-treatment PSA:

RCOG Cure-Rate Data*

PSA Group	*Five-Year Cure-rate*	*Ten-Year Cure-rate*
0.0 – 4.0 ng/ml	96%	85%
4.1 – 10.0 ng/ml	94%	85%
10.1 – 20.0 ng/ml	79%	67%
20.1 ng/ml or more	71%	34%
Overall	89%	72%

*See Appendix 17 for updated data.

RCOG's cure rates were calculated using a post-treatment PSA nadir (the lowest stabilized PSA achieved) of 0.2 ng/ml, the identical PSA nadir used to determine a cure when surgery is the treatment. Also, RCOG had been providing their treatment since 1984.

I interpreted RCOG's data as giving me at least an 85% chance of being cured with their treatment, while this was not 100% (my ideal), this was still a good number.

RCOG's treatment was unique. They had recognized the microscopic cancer cell penetration problem as a major cause of recurring cancer after a treatment. To combat this, their treatment had combined two treatments into one, which they called ProstRcision. ProstRcision— a registered trademark of RCOG— is defined by them as excision of the prostate by irradiation. In concept, this is similar to removal of the prostate by a radical prostatectomy, but no cutting is involved. This greatly minimizes the side effects of impotence and incontinence that are brought about by surgery.

ProstRcision integrates two separate radiation treatments:

1. **Radioactive Seed Implant (Brachytherapy)**
Radioactive seeds are implanted into the prostate gland that delivers radiation for one year.

2. **Precision Conformal Beam Radiation**
Three weeks following the iodine seed implant, conformal beam radiation is delivered to the implanted prostate and seminal vesicles.

Conformal beam and seed radiation are given at the same time, which intensifies the radiation inside the prostate where almost all cancer cells are located. Second, microscopic penetration cancer cells, located outside the prostate capsule and left untreated by the seeds, are treated by the conformal beam part, which irradiates all around the prostate. This synergistic irradiation process provided enough radiation dosage to actually kill all the cancerous and good cells within the prostate gland, thus excising it with the same effect as surgery. This allows ProstRcision to meet the same cure standard as a surgical procedure. There should not be any good, or cancerous, prostate cells remaining after ProstRcision or surgery. To be cured with either treatment, a negligible PSA reading of 0.2 ng/ml, or less, should be achieved and maintained. RCOG's ProstRcision treatment is the only radiation treatment that has adopted the 0.2 ng/ml nadir as a standard cure-rate measure.

RCOG clearly stated in their materials that their practice was not to use hormone therapy as part of their treatment unless the prostate was very enlarged. An important part of the program was the reliance on the post-treatment PSA levels to track how well men were responding to ProstRcision. Administering hormones artificially lowered the post-treatment PSA and reduced the value of this important indicator according to them. RCOG also pointed to studies that showed that hormone therapy did not aid in curing prostate cancer. This seemed to contradict my urologist's suggestion that I begin hormone treatments if I waited more than two weeks to begin treatment.

As I studied ProstRcision, I became more comfortable with the approach. I telephoned to determine how to go about being considered for treatment at RCOG's clinic. They indicated they would send a form that I was to complete, which would allow them to make an assessment of my condition.

Simultaneously, I continued to study other treatments that I thought would address the microscopic penetration problem. I had read Andy Grove's *Fortune* magazine article earlier and decided to go back and study it again. Andy Grove's condition was very similar to mine, he was diagnosed with a PSA of 6.0 (my PSA was 6.4) and he had a Gleason score of 7, which was identical to mine. His 1996 *Fortune* article was very informative, and I realized that, like me, he was most concerned about the potential of cancer recurring after surgery because of the microscopic capsule penetration factor. I studied with a great deal of interest his approach to choosing a treatment, and the treatment he decided on. He chose a treatment that was a variation of the permanent radioactive seed implant. This treatment uses hollow needles that are inserted into the prostate gland through which radioactive seeds containing a higher dose of radiation are temporarily passed through. This temporary seed radiation treatment uses computer guided technology to determine how long the seeds remain within the hollow needles emitting radiation. This treatment, like ProstRcision, is then followed by conformal external beam radiation. In essence, the two treatments seemed very similar with ProstRcision using permanent seed implants and the high-dose-rate (HDR) treatment using temporary seed implants. Knowing that there were at least two treatments aimed specifically at treating the microscopic capsule penetration problem gave me cause for hope.

My urologist's office had arranged an appointment for me to visit the radiation oncology center at Emerson Hospital in my town of Concord. The hospital had recently established a modern center that I understood had some of the newest and best equipment available. For a time, I had served on the Board of Corporators at Emerson Hospital, and I knew a number of the doctors and other medical professionals there. However, this was my first visit to the Radiation Oncology Center. I was greeted by a nurse who was as impressive as the center in the manner in which she greeted me. It was clear they were experienced in dealing with patients who walked through the door suffering from the emotional and psychological pains of cancer.

As I was settled in, I spoke with the oncologist. He examined me and we talked about prostate cancer and radiation treatment. I told him my concerns about external beam radiation alone being a long-term cure for prostate cancer. I indicated that everything I had read pointed to external beam radiation being a follow-up treatment to surgery that failed to remove all the cancer, or used in combination with some form of brachytherapy treatment. This doctor gave me a DRE exam and felt the prostate tumor. The doctor then informed me that Emerson Hospital, in conjunction with Lahey Clinic (about ten miles away), was now providing the HDR treatment! I left the appointment elated. Less than two miles from my house I could get one of the two treatments that would address my biggest fear, microscopic cancer cells penetrating through the prostate gland capsule and into surrounding tissue.

As I left the same medical complex that I had exited just a few days earlier after canceling surgery, I was again struck by what I considered a real gap in prostate care. Here was a treatment available that I didn't know existed locally. Neither my primary care doctor, nor my urologist, counseled me on the availability of this treatment. Where was the medical profession, or specialist, who worked with the prostate cancer patient to help him find the proper treatment? I considered this a form of medical negligence.

This time I was hopeful as I left, but filled with outrage that I came within two days of a surgical treatment that had a 50% chance of failing to cure me of cancer. I became concerned about the lack of a national outrage by men on the state of affairs of prostate cancer treatment.

As a result of my inquiry to RCOG, I received a letter requesting that I submit certain medical records for them to examine to better understand my condition. This information was required before they could accept me for treatment. As I gathered these records, I continued my analysis of the two treatment options that I thought offered the best chance for a complete cure.

RCOG had completed and published a study on the results of their treatment on African Americans. The results showed that the ProstRcision cure rate was the same with African Americans as it was with white men. For me, this was an important study since African American's mortality rate for prostate cancer is among the highest in the world. The reasons for this high mortality rate are not fully understood; however, in choosing a treatment, it was good to know that someone had demonstrated and published results that showed their treatment's ability to normalize this exceedingly high mortality rate.

Dr. Patrick Walsh of Johns Hopkins University is a recognized pioneer in prostate cancer surgical treatment. He pioneered the nerve-sparing procedure, and is credited with having the highest published prostate cancer surgical cure rates in the world. I reviewed a comparison of Dr. Walsh's cure rates with ProstRcision:

Five-Year Cure Rates

PSA Group Before Treatment	RP at Johns Hopkins	ProstRcision at RCOG
0.0 – 4.0 ng/ml	94%	96%
4.1 – 10.0 ng/ml	82%	94%
10.1 – 20.0 ng/ml	72%	79%
20.1 and above	54%	71%
Overall	80%	89%

Ten-Year Cure Rates*

PSA Group Before Treatment	RP at Johns Hopkins	ProstRcision at RCOG
0.0 – 4.0 ng/ml	87%	85%
4.1– 10.0 ng/ml	75%	85%
10.1 – 20.0 ng/ml	30%	67%
20.1 and above	28%	34%
Overall	68%	72%

*See Appendix 17 for updated data.

The cure rates for both treatments are calculated using a PSA nadir of 0.2 ng/ml, thus we are comparing apples to apples. Also, RCOG changed its procedure for implanting the radioactive seeds seven years ago. The data with this new procedure shows an overall seven-year cure rate of 89%, the same as the five-year figure. In

RCOG's literature, they estimate the ten-year, overall cure rate will be no less than 85% when they are able to collect ten-year data using the new procedure. RCOG cites the effect of microscopic capsule penetration as the reason their cure rates are higher then the radical prostatectomy rate (RP); ProstRcision treats this and RP does not.

I also compared the Partin Table data with the failure rates for RP at Johns Hopkins and ProstRcision. I determined the failure rate by subtracting the cure rate from 100%.

Five-Year Results

PSA Group	% with Microsopic Capsule Penetration	Failure Rates	
		RP	ProstRcision
0.0 – 4.0 ng/ml	25%	6%	4%
4.1 – 10.0 ng/ml	50%	18%	6%
10.1 – 20.0 ng/ml	75%	28%	21%
20.1 and above	Almost All	46%	29%

Ten-Year Results

PSA Group	% with Microscopic Capsule Penetration	Failure Rates	
		RP	**ProstRcision**
0.0 – 4.0 ng/ml	25%	13%	15%
4.1 – 10.0 ng/ml	50%	25%	15%
10.1 – 20.0 ng/ml	75%	70%	33%
20.1 and above	Almost All	72%	66%

I performed this analysis to determine if I could find a direct correlation between the microscopic penetration factor and the failure rate for each treatment. The five-year cure-rate data holds up pretty well for each treatment until the 20.1 ng/ml PSA group for RP. The ten-year cure rate is considered to be a more reliable indicator of a complete cure from prostate cancer. Ten years is thought to be enough time for microscopic cancer cells to grow and clearly show a rising PSA and recurring cancer.

The ten-year data shows an almost one for one correlation between the microscopic capsule penetration factor to the failure rate for surgery at the PSA group 10.1 – 20.0. The ProstRcision failure rate remains relatively low until the PSA group 20.1+.

Clearly, neither of these treatments offered what I am sure all prostate cancer patients want, and that is a treatment with a 100% cure rate. However, the more I analyzed RCOG and ProstRcision, the better I felt about their treatment.

One of the major problems in evaluating prostate cancer treatments is that the results of each treatment are based upon the quality of each individual surgeon for surgery, and each individual clinic for radiation treatment. Dr. Walsh's surgical cure rates are the highest published cure rates for the radical prostatectomy (RP) treatment. My urologist never discussed cure rates with me, and I had no idea what they may have been over a five- and ten-year period. However, I had no reason to believe they would have been as good as those published by Dr. Walsh at Johns Hopkins.

I had an appointment to visit a cryosurgery clinic at the University of Massachusetts Medical Center in Worcester, MA. However, it appeared to me that the focus of cryosurgery was to offer an option that would reduce the side effects caused by surgery. I could not find information where cryosurgery addressed microscopic penetration. Also, this procedure didn't have the cure-rate data that was necessary for me to evaluate it's overall cure-rate effectiveness. I decided to cancel my cryosurgery appointment and focus on my radiation options.

Standard brachytherapy treatment (permanent seed implant without any form of external beam radiation) is also offered in the Boston area. My study of this treatment showed that it was also an alternative to surgery that focused on treating cancer within the prostate gland without any treatment of microscopic penetration. For my condition, I also dismissed this treatment as being inadequate. In addition, brachytherapy had a history that was problematic for me. It seemed that this treatment was hailed as a major breakthrough in the 1970's when thousands of men chose it over surgery considering it less invasive and offering a chance of cure. Based on my research, the results were disastrous and thousands of men died after having this treatment. Some accounts that I read called this one of the major medical disasters in history.

The old brachytherapy procedure relied upon a retropubic surgical procedure to implant the radioactive seed directly into the prostate gland. A new approach to implanting the radioactive seed, perineally, where the seeds are implanted inside thin needles through the skin of the perineum (the area between the scrotum and anus) is now used. This procedure uses ultrasonic guided needles to properly place the seeds inside the prostate gland for a uniform radiation field. This new approach is widely used to provide brachytherapy treatment throughout the United States. But as with surgery, the quality of this treatment is directly related to the skill and quality of the individual treatment provider. Even if this treatment were an option for me, I would need to look at hard data on the cure rates of the provider, which would probably not be available for most.

It appeared to me that my options for treatment were ProstRcision in Atlanta, GA, and HDR within two miles of my house. I began to feel lucky to have a treatment option so close to home. With the HDR, or "Smart Bomb" treatment as it is sometimes referred, I would be in the clinic overnight for only one night and able to stop by the radiation center on my way to, or from, the office each day. In essence, there would be no disruption of my life to obtain this treatment. RCOG had made it clear that all radiation treatments after the seed implant would have to be performed by them in Atlanta. Clearly, I was leaning toward the HDR treatment. What remained for me was to analyze their cure rates and other data.

I told Juarez that I had all but decided to have the HDR treatment but I wanted her to accompany me on one last visit with the doctor at Lahey Clinic. She was insistent that I still send all of my records to RCOG.

Prior to my appointment, I went on the Internet to obtain some additional data on HDR. It was not easy finding access to the center that pioneered this treatment in Seattle. However, I was able to find it and eventually placed a telephone call to the center to speak with someone. I obtained a telephone message that simply stated that they were not accepting any new patients at this time. My interest was not in going to Seattle for treatment, but to obtain some data on HDR treatment results. However, this avenue proved fruitless and I would just have to wait until I met with the doctor here.

Juarez and I made our very short journey to the clinic to meet with the doctor for some final discussion on HDR. We sat down with him and began a discussion on the procedure. After a short time, I decided I really needed to get my questions answered on their cure-rate data and other statistics before we went much further.

I asked the doctor what the cure rates were. He thought for a moment and answered, 100%. How can that be? I asked. I have never seen any data suggesting that any treatment offered a 100% cure rate. The doctor was very open and honest with me. He simply said that his clinic had not been providing this treatment long enough to have any failures. Well, I clearly understood what he was saying and told him that under the circumstances, I could not choose to have this treatment. I had tried to obtain cure-rate data from three centers that provided this treatment and I was unable to do so.

I left the clinic very disappointed, and with Georgia on my mind. It appeared that with all of its inconveniences, Georgia was where I could find the treatment that offered me the best chance for a cure. Again, I thought about this situation and found it somewhat amusing. How could I ever explain to the folks in Massachusetts that Georgia offers a better treatment for prostate cancer?

I spoke with the doctors at RCOG. They had evaluated my medical records and thought I was a good candidate for their treatment. In speaking with the doctor at RCOG and getting additional information in the mail, I determined that they had a unique approach in providing their treatment, an approach that had proven itself over time. Also, RCOG regularly published their data and the results of studies that they performed on their data collected from patients for peer review. I had studied as many of their responses as I could find and was very comfortable with their treatment approach.

In RCOG's treatment plan for me, I also learned something new about my condition. The maximum external beam radiation that they provide is administered over a seven-week period and they had prescribed the maximum load for me because my Gleason score was 7. They administer both six- and seven-week external beam radiation programs. If a patient's PSA is less than 10 and his Gleason is less than 7, he'll receive the six-week program. If his PSA is 10 and above, or his Gleason score is 7 or above, then he'll receive the seven-week program. The seven-week program is designed for what RCOG considers a larger probability of microscopic capsule penetration spread. What had frightened me most about my condition, the 50% probability of microscopic capsule penetration, was worse than I thought. Using the Partin Table data alone, I had not factored in the Gleason score of 7. Luckily, I had found a treatment that compensated for this factor.

I made my decision for treatment at RCOG in Atlanta, GA, after weeks of intensive gathering of data and analysis. Over this period of time, my priority was finding a treatment that I thought would cure my prostate cancer. I didn't have the benefit of any objective advice from a medical care specialist. I was on my own. I only spoke with doctors providing the various treatment services, but I had to make the final choice. My urologist never called to see how I was progressing. This had been a very lonely time but my battle plan was now firmly in place.

A divine twist of fate became apparent when I received my treatment instructions from RCOG. In bold letters on my instructions were printed:

ATTENTION ALL IMPLANT PATIENTS
If you are taking Glucophage for diabetes you must stop these medications at least 4 to 5 days before implant

I immediately thought back to that morning when I met the stranger in the donut shop. Not only had he led me to the discovery of my prostate cancer, but he had also led me to an approach of managing my diabetes that eliminated my dependence on Glucophage and a conflict with my chosen treatment.

After selecting a prostate cancer treatment and prior to beginning the treatment, I had time to reflect on the medical system that I was in the midst of.

Chapter VI
Silence and A System Flawed

It became quickly evident during my analysis that, in relative silence, men are engaged in a raging battle with prostate cancer. With 200,000 plus men diagnosed each year and 30,000 deaths, the havoc that prostate cancer causes can best be understood when compared to other incidences of human devastation. The 47,000 combat deaths that US servicemen and women sustained in Vietnam is one such incidence. However, consider that these 47,000 combat deaths were inflicted over the 15-year duration of America's longest war, while approximately 500,000 men were dying from prostate cancer. Since the end of the Vietnam War casualties, another 1,000,000 U.S. men have been prostate cancer casualties. Another example of prostate cancer devastation is seen when compared with the approximately 27,000 men, women, and children who are killed in automobile accidents each year. Automobile safety issues are visible everywhere, every day, and, needless to say, the Vietnam War held news headlines throughout its 15-year duration. On the other hand, little attention has been given to the plight of men battling prostate cancer. Maybe we need to dramatize prostate cancer deaths with body bag counts, or post the casualties on billboards, a practice in some cities for automobile accidents. Whatever approach we take, the silence that we have witnessed for years is counterproductive and it is a silence that kills.

In my opinion, this silence has fostered a system without oversight or accountability—a system that is seriously flawed at every level. To receive prostate cancer care and treatment, men must navigate this flawed system, much the same way combat troops would navigate a mine field. Men must succumb to the treatment recommendation of urologists, who have a vested interested in their treatment service or, men must find and evaluate other treatment options usually in an emotional and sometime defenseless state of mind.

In a weakened emotional state, I initially succumbed to my urologist's recommendation, but reversed my decision and sought other treatment options. In fact, I never spoke to my urologist again after our last meeting. To this day, I have received no guidance or note of concern for my condition from the prostate cancer medical specialist whom I was referred to by my primary care doctor. While I considered him my prostate cancer doctor, he clearly viewed himself as offering a service that I declined. I have found that my case is the norm and not the exception, when men decline the radical prostatectomy service that urologists provide, or any treatment service provided by other specialists.

My introduction to prostate care began in February, 1994, at age 51, when I had my first PSA test and digital rectal examination (DRE). The PSA test results were 3.3 and the DRE was normal. My record listed the next PSA result in 1996 when it was measured at 4.1. The DRE was normal. My next PSA test, according to my record, was not until 1999 when it measured 5.8 and, again, the DRE was considered normal. In March 2000, my PSA went to 6.4 and I was referred to a urologist and diagnosed with prostate cancer.

Based on my research, I now know that I had a prostate problem in 1994. With a PSA of 3.3 at age 51, something bad was happening within my prostate gland, especially when considering that I am in two of the highest risk groups—I am African American and I have a family history of prostate cancer.

My experience in 1994 highlights the major flaw within the prostate care system: the general lack of awareness and knowledge of prostate problems among men and primary care doctors.

I had no knowledge about the prostate and related problems when I had my first PSA test. I didn't know that I was in a high-risk group, and since the doctor told me I was fine, I didn't question his findings. Considering that men will receive tests for the prostate for as much as 50% of their lifetime, awareness of the prostate and problems associated with it are almost totally lacking among men. I believe this can be attributed to a system that has not yet reconciled itself to whether early and routine PSA screening is needed and has not aggressively reached out to educate men about prostate care.

When considering that the headquarters for the Centers for Disease Control (CDC) and the American Cancer Society are both located in Atlanta, Georgia (literally across the street from each other), and they take opposing views on early PSA screenings, then there is an inherent problem that impacts education and awareness efforts. This is symbolized by the physical closeness and philosophical differences of these organizations.

The American Cancer Society advocates early and routine screening and the CDC does not. Because there is no consensus among medical organizations, there appears to be no leadership or oversight that is forcing a definitive message to general practitioners who are the first line of defense against prostate problems. In fact, the American Association of Family Practitioners and the American Society of Internal Medicine do not advocate routine screening for prostate cancer. This makes me question whether family practitioners are properly trained and philosophically in tune with the important role they play in prostate care. For the most part, primary care doctors adhere to a guideline that the prostate is fine as long as the PSA is under 4.0. This general guideline makes no exception for high risk groups or how fast the PSA is rising, and most importantly, the age when a man approaches the 4.0 threshold.

Based on my experience and analysis, I do not believe that general practitioners are equipped to provide proper prostate care, beginning with PSA testing and the DRE. This state of affairs is coupled with the lack of an awareness program that would equip men with enough knowledge to perform some self-diagnosis. Consequently, there is a critical flaw at the very beginning of prostate care, and I personally suffered because of it. How does it reveal itself now that I have been diagnosed with cancer? According to all statistics that I have seen, the cure rate for cancer treated with a PSA of 4.0 or less is higher than my pretreatment PSA of 6.4, and this fact holds true for every man.

The fact is, every man's PSA will move through the 4.0 level if it goes higher. A strong awareness campaign could dramatically increase the number of men diagnosed with cancer at the lower PSA levels, thereby increasing their chances of a treatment cure. When you are talking about life and death, every single percentage point in your favor is critical.

I considered my primary care physician a good doctor. He had been my family's doctor for more than twenty years. However, I now know that he was not competent in meeting my prostate care needs. I do not blame him. I consider a medical system that does not realize a prostate care specialist is needed for men, at fault. This, in my opinion, is the biggest flaw within a seriously flawed system. Within the current system, men have no doctor to examine and advise them on prostate care. We are poorly examined by general practitioners and usually when our lives are visibly at risk, we are transitioned to a urologist. My father, who was raised on a North

Carolina farm, often characterized this type of predicament as "caught between a rock and a hard place."

I vividly remember prostate examinations in my doctor's office. They consisted of extracting blood for a PSA test and a digital rectal examination (DRE). Never once, over twenty years that I visited my doctor, did we have a conversation about the prostate or potential prostate problems. This may have been OK, had he understood how to read the PSA results relative to my prostate cancer risk group, or known the best techniques for administering a DRE. I use my doctor as an example only because I know he represents a position common among many general practitioners.

I understand that the PSA test has only been available and relied upon since the late 1980's or early 1990's; however, many general practitioners today do not know how to use it as a prostate cancer diagnostic tool. In fact, after I was diagnosed with prostate cancer and set out to find a treatment alone, I continually interfaced with my general practitioner (which was only necessary for insurance purposes.) After a while, he confided that I knew more about prostate cancer than most doctors. I took this as a compliment for my amateur research efforts, I certainly hoped this wasn't true. Sadly, very sadly, I believe he was being honest with me. For men, this is a frightening indictment of our medical care system, but a reality.

A prostate care specialist—a doctor knowledgeable about the most current testing, analysis, research, and treatments available to guide me along the proper prostate cancer route—would have made an enormous difference. Such a specialist would have immediately suspected a problem with my first PSA reading in 1994, knowing that I was in a high-risk group for prostate cancer. As my PSA continued to rise rapidly, this specialist would have noted the PSA velocity to be too high and ordered the proper test to pinpoint my cancer earlier. Had my cancer escaped detection until my 1999 PSA, which measured 5.8, this specialist certainly would not have sent me home to wait three months for another test. I sincerely believe that I had prostate cancer for at least six years before it was detected by the current system.

Doctors rely upon the DRE to literally "feel" the tumor on the prostate gland with their finger. This is not a pleasant examination. I haven't spoken to a single man who wants the "finger." Though we have learned to bear the "finger," it is a very inexact examination. My doctor never once felt a problem with my prostate. However, the very first examination that I received when I was referred to the urologist was an ultrasound (TRUS–transrectal ultrasound) of the prostate gland. Within five minutes, the urologist told me that he saw a problem on the right side of my prostate gland.

The prostate care specialist I envision would eliminate or supplement the DRE with ultrasound readings of the prostate gland. Why don't doctors use this diagnostic tool now as opposed to the DRE? If there is a problem with the prostate, the prostate care specialist will perform the biopsy, and if cancer is present, stage the cancer.

Knowing the various treatment options, the prostate care specialist will advise men on the best treatments available to them based on their cancer stage. This specialist will not provide any treatments directly, but have the responsibility of working with the patient in a supportive role as he is treated for cancer. I have not seen, or even heard of this much-needed prostate care specialist during my experience.

Men now are handed off from the general practitioner to a urologist for a prostate gland biopsy when a problem is suspected. From this point forward, men are at the mercy of a doctor whose advice, at best, is suspect if you are diagnosed with cancer. In today's system, the urologist performs the biopsy and if it is positive, stages the cancer and primarily recommends surgery. Men have little or no recourse to question either the diagnosis or the treatment. Once again, men are "caught between a rock and a hard place."

During the past ten years, a great deal of work has been done by the medical community in developing and evaluating new treatments. Some of the treatments are proving themselves to be viable and some are not. However, many urologists are not familiar with what is happening within their own field any more than general practitioners. Therefore, they can only recommend what they know.

If a man dares not to accept the urologist's recommendation and begins to explore and evaluate other treatment options, then he is faced with the difficult job of gathering information, understanding it, and finally making a treatment decision. Most men are either not capable or willing to take on this task, nor should they be required to. As a minimum, in the absence of a prostate care specialist, the current system should require some standardization.

It is unbelievable to me that there is no oversight of prostate cancer treatments that I have been able to identify other than what is imposed by the medical profession itself—very little! What does this mean?

1. Doctors are free to recommend and provide any treatment they want regardless of the cancer's stage or any other condition. Most doctors will recommend the specific treatment they provide.

2. Doctors do not have to inform men of their individual cure-rate success and usually do not.

3. There are no universal standards of cure-rate measurements across treatments and, therefore, no direct way to compare different treatments on an "apples to apples" basis.

Just these factors alone make it almost impossible for most men to deviate from their original urologist's recommendation. Most men are trapped inside this flawed system with their lives in the hands of doctors with vested business interests in their individual treatments. Men are easy prey in this system and it is not unusual to hear stories of men having a radical prostatectomy with a PSA in excess of 20 with no follow-up radiation treatment. There literally is no oversight or accountability within the present system and some of the stories I have heard from men are absolutely outrageous. For example, I spoke with a man whose PSA had tested at 15+ for more than two years. He was urinating frequently, a clear sign of trouble. His urologist had given him a biopsy but found no cancer. I asked about the number of biopsy needles, he didn't seem to know. I asked if his urologist had performed a "percent free PSA" analysis, he had never heard of this. His urologist had, however, recommended a radical prostatectomy to eliminate his frequent urinary problems!

The urologist would subject this 70+ year old man to the complications of surgery and the possibility of urinary incontinence after having found no cancer. This, to me, is a ludicrous approach to solving a problem that is much easier to live with than the potential side effects of surgery. This urologist should have ordered the proper tests to determine if the man did indeed have cancer.

While the existing system fails most men in some way, it is especially harsh on African Americans. I believe system failures account for the mortality disparity between white Americans and African Americans. There are rumors that African Americans typically have a more aggressive form of prostate cancer than white Americans. I have not seen any data or information to support this. What we do know is that African Americans prostate cancer incidence rate is 60% higher than white Americans and the mortality rate is 140% higher. African Americans are placed, as a category, in a high-risk group. Since the system does not detect cancer early enough in African Americans, and knowing that the treatment cure rate is directly related to early detection, the mortality rate difference is easy to see.

Using the data published by Dr. Patrick Walsh on his 10-year cure rates for men receiving radical prostatectomy (RP) treatment at Johns Hopkins, will help illustrate this point.

PSA Group Before Treatment	RP Cure rate at Johns Hopkins	Corresponding Failure Rate
0.0 – 4.0	87%	13%
4.1 – 10.0	75%	25%
10.1 – 20.0	30%	70%
20.1 or more	28%	72%

This data clearly shows a nearly 2:1 failure rate between pretreatment PSA groups (0.0 – 4.0) and (4.1 – 10.0) and almost a 3:1 failure rate difference between pretreatment PSA groups (4.1 – 10.0) and (10.1 – 20.0). Even with the current flawed system, good medical care will detect prostate cancer much earlier than poor medical care. It is well known that African American health care, overall, is not up to the standards of white America. The lack of prostate cancer awareness, early screening and treatment alone could account for the mortality disparity between

African Americans and white Americans—a situation that can be remedied.

I should also emphasize that not all doctors are equal in the quality of treatment they provide. Dr. Walsh has the highest published cure rates for prostate cancer when surgery is the treatment. In addition, should external beam radiation be the treatment of choice for the higher PSA levels, then the cure rates are even lower. The type and quality of treatment at whatever stage it is administered is thus a major factor in mortality rates. Also, not all treatments even offer a chance for long-term cure. I have talked with men on hormone treatments as their first and primary treatment, and I always wonder whether they know that this treatment is not a potential cure for prostate cancer even though it may lower the PSA.

To combat the exceedingly high mortality rates among African Americans, the first approach by many is to increase the level of PSA screening in African American communities. On the surface, this would appear to be the proper move, but the problem is much more complex and requires significantly more attention and effort.

African American men are diagnosed with approximately 25,000 new cases of prostate cancer each year, accounting for approximately 37% of all cancers diagnosed among African American men. This exceeds the estimated 22,000 cases of HIV/AIDS reported annually for African American men, women, and children. According to American Cancer Society data, African Americans are diagnosed with prostate cancer at an earlier age with the incidence rate of African Americans at the 60 to 64 age group, almost equal to the incidence rate for white Americans in the 70 to 74 age group. The five-year survival rate for African Americans is 75% yet 90% for white Americans. However, according to data published by the American Cancer

Society the five-year survival rate is 100% when cancer is diagnosed at a local stage, 94% when diagnosed at a regional stage, and 31% when diagnosed at a distant stage (cancer has metastasized). These statistics indicate that African Americans are typically diagnosed when the cancer is more advanced. All of this data points to a system that is flawed to the point of negligence for African Americans.

Increased education and awareness are critical for African Americans. The American Cancer Society and National Comprehensive Cancer Network (NCCN) recommends PSA screening begin at age 45 for high-risk groups. African Americans are designated as a high-risk group! By definition, African Americans need to be educated about the prostate at a much earlier age, beginning at age 40. At age 45 and above, I believe, African American men need to know their PSA number as well as they know their weight! Since the cancer incidence rate appears to be ten years sooner for African Americans, then it is logical to begin PSA testing ten years earlier. The prostate care system must be overhauled to be responsive to this urgent need among African Americans. There is enough need for leadership in this health crisis for community leaders and all other leaders to take part in this education and awareness initiative. Personally, I never knew that I should begin PSA testing earlier than 50 years of age, and I doubt that many African Americans are aware of this either. When I got my first PSA test at 51, I thought I was within the time frame established for all men to begin PSA testing.

Prostate care specialists are critical to meeting the needs in African American communities. Since prostate cancer is detected at earlier ages, then treatments that offer the very best chance for a complete cure are needed by this high-risk group. Otherwise, a very long and costly journey of ongoing, life-long treatments will be required.

Again, prostate cancer is curable if it is caught early, and the correct treatment is selected.

The prostate care system today is intercepting African Americans at a later stage in life when it must intercede at an earlier age than white Americans. PSA screening campaigns, without the early education and awareness programs, and prostate care counseling will not fix this problem. In fact, many PSA screening campaigns become feeder systems for urologists. The urologist is not necessarily going to provide the counseling and guidance that men need and that will lead to a prostate cancer cure and a reduction in mortality rates. The urologist is likely to recommend surgery as the "gold standard" treatment, as was done for me.

Where do we get leadership and the oversight needed to make the prostate care system responsive in the United States? Men must take on prostate cancer with the intent of forcing the needed changes within the medical care system. But this is not just a battle for men; our wives, mothers, sisters and daughters all suffer when we suffer, and our sons are at risk. This is a challenge for the entire family. This is not a battle over ideology; again, prostate cancer is curable if detected early enough. The medical profession is capable of providing the treatments necessary for cure, if the cancer is caught soon enough. There has to be leadership that forces the system to be as good as it can be for all men.

Oversight is another issue. With nearly 30,000 men dying each year and another 100,000+ receiving some form of treatment, prostate cancer is a serious public health issue. Where is government oversight in this equation? How can federal and state government agencies stay out of this battle?

Today, men are forced to shop for prostate cancer treatment as if shopping for an automobile or some other commodity. However, there are no standards that allow men to compare the various treatment options on an equal basis relative to their effectiveness in offering a cure. Each treatment specialist gives you their cure rate sometimes, and sometimes they refuse. Suppose you were purchasing an automobile and could not obtain the miles per gallon, engine size or other performance parameters, but you were told it would drive fine. This is the typical situation we are faced with when shopping for prostate cancer treatment cure-rate data. When we are able to obtain this data, it is often stated in different measurement units. This is analogous to having an automobile fuel consumption stated as 50 per gallon and not knowing whether this is 50 miles per gallon, or 50 kilometers per gallon, or 50 inches per gallon.

With automobile safety, government standards exist for almost every facet, yet the yearly deaths from automobile accidents have never equaled those resulting from prostate cancer. The government needs to insist on standardization of treatment cure-rate measurement, and disclosure by doctors of their individual cure rates according to these standards. Today, the public has no way to differentiate between the results of Dr. Frank Critz of RCOG and Dr. Walsh of Johns Hopkins and a storefront urologist performing surgeries. Because the storefront urologist is not required to disclose his treatment success data it will typically not be available. Some men asked their urologists about their cure-rate data and were told by the urologist that they were surgeons, not researchers.

Men need help to change this flawed system. We need to create a system where men understand, at an early age, that their prostate can be a source of problems and even cause for death. We need to have a place to go where a specialist can help us evaluate the health of our individual prostates, and advise us on what to do if we detect a problem. We need a way to quickly understand the right treatment for our cancer when we are diagnosed. We need the best opportunity to cure our cancer and move on with our lives. All these things are possible today, once we change the current system with its built-in vested interest for the doctors who administer it, to a system that is responsive to the needs of men facing the deadly prostate cancer disease.

In reality, the current system is the same dark and silent closet that we have chosen for our prostate cancer suffering. However, it is the flawed medical system of today that I, and countless others, have struggled to navigate.

Chapter VII
Independence Day 2000

When I was growing up in North Carolina, the Fourth of July was a day when we would typically go fishing early in the morning, and later to a community baseball game with lots of hot dogs, followed by firecrackers. In my small community, this day was filled with lighthearted fun and excitement. Living in Concord, MA, for the past 20 years, where the shot was fired to start the American Revolution, July 4th has had a very different meaning.

The Concord community works diligently to give this day its true symbolic purpose. Early each July 4th morning, since I have lived in Concord, the Concord Minutemen march by my street waking me to the sound of their drums. I don't believe there is a more historically conscious town in the United States than Concord. Not much has changed in my town since the shot was fired that propelled this nation to its independence. I have come to enjoy and appreciate this very unique town and Fourth of July festivities. However, this July 4th would forever change this day's meaning for me.

On Independence Day 2000, Juarez and I boarded an airplane and headed for Atlanta, GA and the beginning of my physical battle with this killer. After all of my agonizing struggles to get to this point, I was now ready to fire my first real shot. July 4th seemed a fitting day to begin my journey to reclaim my health.

As the plane flew over Boston, I still felt it odd that I had to make this trip to receive, what I considered, the best treatment available for a prostate cancer cure. When I was first diagnosed, I never envisioned such a scenario. I was thankful for having this option, but I was also saddened that this treatment was not available to the countless number of men who could benefit from it, but who wouldn't have the opportunity to make this trip.

Atlanta seemed exceptionally hot as we arrived. I was accustomed to hot summer days in the south, but this was a blistering day. Maybe being away from the South had made me more sensitive to the heat. I immediately began to ask myself how I was going to survive Atlanta during the middle of summer.

I have relatives and a number of friends in Atlanta, but Juarez, my sister, and I had decided that we would not let family members there know of my condition. Our concern was for my mother. At a time when she had not recovered from my father's death, we didn't want her to have to face questions each day from her friends about my health and explain to them why I was in Atlanta. In fact, she had her own serious questions and concerns as to why it was necessary for me to be there.

We checked into the Hyatt, downtown. After we got settled, we began to think about how we were going to celebrate this holiday alone in Atlanta. We really didn't have any idea what was going on in this city, so we drove to Buckhead to find a place for dinner. We decided on the Palm Restaurant, since there was a Palm Restaurant in Boston that Juarez and I enjoyed. We were lucky to find a table on the patio where a band played. We had been taking our time eating and enjoying the band when we noticed a crowd beginning to gather on a grassy area across the street from the restaurant. Our waitress let us know that people were gathering for the fireworks. By pure luck, we had found ourselves right in the center of where the fireworks display would take place later that evening. So we relaxed, continued to enjoy the band, and watched the fireworks. We had chosen not to focus our time together on the impending treatment. Our spirits were lifted.

As we awoke the next morning, it was time to get down to business and map out our route to Decatur and Radiotherapy Clinics of Georgia. I was really anxious to see this facility that I had selected, primarily over the Internet, to fight the battle of my life. I had seen their facilities on the brochure they sent, but I was always skeptical about brochure pictures compared to reality. I guess this is what people go through with on-line dating, I thought.

My implant procedure was scheduled for the next day, July 6th. My appointment with RCOG was in the afternoon so Juarez and I decided to scout around the beltway and locate the implant outpatient facility before going to RCOG. RCOG uses the outpatient services of hospitals and clinics for the implant procedure and provides the daily radiation treatment at their clinics. I was dumbfounded by the Atlanta beltway traffic, which rivaled the chaos in Boston. This was preventing me from finding my destination and it was becoming frustrating.

We eventually found our way to RCOG. There it was, just as it appeared in the brochure, a brick Georgia facility. I was now face-to-face with my hope for beating prostate cancer.

As we entered RCOG we saw men seated in the various areas. There was a relatively large area with computers, reading materials, coffee, and it seemed to be quite busy. I noted that the men were in relatively good spirits as they talked with each other. No one seemed ill. I wasn't sure what I had expected entering RCOG. My evaluation had been so very analytically detailed that at this point, I wasn't even sure that I had ever thought about the fact that I was going to a medical facility where they would be treating men with cancer. I hadn't really considered being around men who were sick from radiation. No, my focus had strictly been on understanding the treatment and its cure rate over a long enough period that I could evaluate it. But, this was real, and I was happy that I didn't see anyone looking deathly ill from this treatment. On the contrary, they looked fine. They were smiling and talking. At about this time, I was called in to meet my doctor.

I was assigned to Dr. James Benton and we went to an examining area where he reviewed my records and talked about the ProstRcision treatment. Well, by then, I had been pretty familiar with ProstRcision and I was anxious to get on with things. After a short discussion, he asked me to prepare for a DRE. I thought I was finished with the DRE's. I'd never spoken to a single man who liked these examinations. Upon performing the DRE, Dr. Benton was able to find the tumor on the prostate gland. He seemed a little perplexed that my primary care doctor hadn't detected it earlier. Dr. Benton was the third doctor over the past three months to give me a DRE, and I noticed that they each had a different technique and was beginning to understand how one doctor could detect an irregularity and another would not.

After a lengthy discussion with Dr. Benton, wherein he told me that Dr. Hamilton Williams would do the implant, Juarez and I left RCOG and headed back into the city for the evening to prepare for implant surgery the next day. We had been provided with instructions for a cleansing procedure that included no food or drink, and a self-administered enema. The battle was about ready to begin and I was getting psyched. At last, I thought, at last I could do something about this killer.

The day had finally arrived. It was a typical hot July day in Atlanta as Juarez and I drove out to the implant service center. We arrived and sat for awhile before I was called to begin the preparations.

I put on the gown that the nurses provided for me. Prior to the blood pressure test, the nurse cautioned me that my reading would probably be above normal because of the anxiety that I was under. I assured the nurse that I only felt a sense of relief by being there. After my readings were taken, I think the nurse was shocked to see how normal they were. However, as I waited to go into the operating room, I noticed that three different attendants, or nurses, stopped by to check on me and to ask me what seemed to be the same set of questions concerning my readiness as they reviewed the readings. At last I was wheeled into the operating room.

The brochure that I had received from RCOG depicted this surgical procedure being performed by two doctors. I never asked any questions specifically about this procedure, but when I was taken into the operating room, I noticed quite a crowd of people clad in caps and gowns who appeared like they were going to be involved in something. As I looked around, I asked one of them if I was the only patient in the room, and he answered, yes. I felt a little alarmed. I then asked how many people were in there, as I was being surrounded by what appeared to be an army. He looked around and answered, ten. Ten! What were they all going to do?

When I awoke, I noticed only one thing—the presence of a catheter in my penis that was painful and very uncomfortable. A nurse explained that the catheter would stay in overnight, and be removed the next morning. I immediately began the countdown.

I was wheeled into a recovery area and after about an hour, I was able to get up. Juarez and I drove back to the hotel.

One hundred and twelve radioactive iodine seeds were permanently implanted into my prostate gland. I was trying to coexist with this damn catheter for one night. If I had had surgery, the catheter would have to remain in for three weeks after leaving the hospital—about four weeks total. That alone, I figured, was enough reason not to have surgery.

After a very restless night, morning finally arrived and I was up bright and early and ready to go back to RCOG to get the catheter removed. I didn't notice anything or anyone. I had only one thought on my mind. When I went to the receptionist's desk, the receptionist looked at me and said, "Oh, you must be here to have your catheter removed." I was sure they could see the pained look in my eyes.

After a while, I was finally called back. The attendant placed me on a table. I didn't feel much pain as she removed the tube from my penis. I was thankful RCOG had a delicate person perform this procedure. Immediately, I gained some added respect for RCOG. Brilliant people, I thought.

While I was in for the catheter removal, the same attendant began a series of simulation procedures to prepare me for the external beam radiation treatment, which was to begin in three weeks. She finished quickly, completing that phase of my treatment.

After the catheter removal, I felt like a new man. Juarez smiled as she saw the relief on my face. We left RCOG and decided to have a day in the city. We had lunch and went to see a movie. We ended my first day of recovery with dinner, and toasted a successful beginning in my battle with prostate cancer.

On Saturday, July 8th, we boarded a plane and headed back to Boston.

Chapter VIII
Battling Prostate Cancer

Back in Boston, I was in the office every day for three weeks without any complications from the implant. Although I was prescribed pain medication, I didn't need to take a single pill. The one issue that I had to deal with was getting up three times during the night to go to the bathroom. The doctors at RCOG had aptly warned me that this would be a side effect. The needles that were inserted in the prostate gland to implant the radioactive seeds caused swelling, which disrupted the normal urinary flow.

During the time that I was home, I was finally able to remove myself from any worries about treatment. With the beginning of treatment, my transition from fear of cancer to focusing on a cure was a psychological rebirth. I was able, again, to look toward the future and feel a renewed strength and energy in my battle. I had done everything in my power to select the best treatment available for a cure, now it was out of my hands completely. I was turning my treatment over to the medical team I had selected and praying for God's continued blessings.

Three weeks passed quickly and I began preparing to go back to Atlanta for the seven-week external beam treatment phase. Juarez wanted to go back with me, but I tried to assure her that I would be OK alone for a while.

When I entered the lobby at RCOG, ten to fifteen men were seated throughout the various seating areas. We introduced ourselves and began to discuss various aspects of our treatment stages. Individual radiation treatments were scheduled for six or seven weeks depending upon the stage of cancer. My treatment was scheduled for seven. As we introduced ourselves, I was struck by two factors: first, men were here from all parts of the United States and other countries, and second, their spirits, under the circumstances were high. These were not men consumed by fear, but men of hope. Indeed, our common journey had placed us here together, a place that we would make home during this hot summer. Our common bond of battling cancer allowed us to interact freely and openly.

I had met Dan Graham and his wife, Cindy, during the implant treatment phase. They were from Milwaukee, Wisconsin. I recognized them in the lobby and we started a conversation. Dan and I had brought our golf clubs and were interested in locating nearby golf courses. As we talked, other men joined in and soon we had a group of golfers. We had golf set up before we took our first radiation treatment. Why not? No one appeared sick or frightened about the battle we faced. Prostate cancer at first is silent, as silent as the men it invades. A man may not even know he is sick. However, when it has moved into place throughout the body, prostate cancer brings with it such havoc that it is difficult to get back to a safe harbor. Luckily, all the men had detected this storm soon enough to fight it, with a good chance of winning and everyone seemed up for the battle.

Most of the men had applied for housing at the Hope Lodge. I had visited this facility on my first trip down and it appeared to be a comfortable and interesting housing concept created especially for cancer patients from out of town. However, it was fully occupied and most of us had to find nearby housing and wait for an opening.

I had gotten settled into a comfortable suite hotel only a ten-minute drive from RCOG. Some of the other men were scattered close by in similar hotels, others had been moved directly into the Hope Lodge.

It was time to focus on RCOG treatments. This was my very first experience with any type of medical treatment and I really didn't know what to expect. What type of people would I be interacting with? Doctors? My recent experience with doctors gave me some concerns as to how RCOG's doctors might interact with their patients. What was the culture of this clinic? All of these were issues going through my mind as I prepared to begin this daily treatment phase. Again, I evaluated treatments based on their data and information. All these were factors that I could not evaluate analytically. I would have to experience them.

I met with Dr. Benton and he went over the treatment procedures with me in detail. I was allotted a time for daily radiation treatments. Each treatment would last only a few minutes, after which I would be free to go and do whatever I pleased until my appointment the next day. There were questionnaires that I had to complete every Monday prior to treatment that would allow the doctors to monitor any effects the radiation was having on urination, sexual function, and the rectum. Dr. Benton indicated that doctors at RCOG reviewed these questionnaires as a team in monitoring the radiation treatment and any problems that might occur. Dr. Benton also told me that I might suffer some fatigue as a result of the treatments, but the most noticeable side effect would be urinary problems. I was told to expect a weak urinary stream and plan to get up a lot at night.

I also learned that RCOG had scheduled weekly seminars dealing with prostate care and prostate cancer. A dinner would be served prior to each seminar. In addition, they held a weekly nutritional workshop. RCOG had, in fact, put together a rather full schedule of activities, it seemed. I was getting a little concerned about my golfing plans.

As treatment began, I was introduced to the radiation technicians responsible for administering the daily treatments. This was a committed group of specialists who were pleasant and made treatments enjoyable as best they could. I didn't see how they could possibly take a single additional patient. Also, I was amazed at the number of men from seemingly all parts of the United States, Canada, and other countries. RCOG, indeed had been discovered.

At our very first group seminar, an orientation, all the men present introduced themselves and told us where they came from. A RCOG doctor, Dr. Williams, then asked those referred by their urologist to raise their hands. Startlingly, not a single hand was raised! Dr. Williams said this was usually the case. He told us we were a very unique group of men, and while we might not recognize that initially, we would over time. Most men who chose RCOG, he said, came from the ranks of those who could research and analyze information and make a decision based on this analysis, which often ran counter to the medical advice they may have been receiving.

After a week, I was able to get into the swing of the treatments. In fact, I was learning to enjoy the camaraderie. All the doctors at RCOG were easily accessible, including Dr. Frank Critz, the founder of the clinic. They were active in the seminar series and available to answer questions.

RCOG introduced us to an "Integrated Prostate Health Plan," which was the subject of one of their seminars. This plan focused on eating properly and was the introduction to their dietary workshops. Other seminars gave us a thorough understanding of the prostate, prostate cancer and RCOG's treatment history and philosophy. The RCOG seminar series was the type of education and awareness program that men needed earlier in life and prior to being diagnosed with cancer. This program was well conceived and presented. It gave us an opportunity to interact with doctors at RCOG in a group setting, which facilitated our education and knowledge. I learned more about the prostate and prostate cancer from these sessions than I had ever expected to know.

The daily treatments at Radiotherapy Clinics of Georgia were straightforward. There was no pain and very few side effects. The doctors and staff really tried to make treatment as joyful as anything that any of us could have ever imagined. While I was impressed with the Clinic when I made my choice for their treatment, I became more impressed each day. The other men all seemed to share the same opinion.

The treatments employed very sophisticated conformal beam techniques to enhance a cure and to minimize side effects. My discussions with the doctors for other treatment options never touched on the procedures used here. Now I clearly understood why the Radiotherapy Clinics would not simply perform the implant and let me receive the external beam radiation at a hospital at home as I, and many of the other men, had requested.

The computer operations for planning the seed implant for each patient was located next to the radiation area. Being somewhat inquisitive, I went into this area and began a conversation. I was able to view some of the computerized planning and mapping of the radiation fields generated by the implanted iodine seeds. This was an impressive operation and it gave me a good insight into the precise nature of the ProstRcision treatment.

After a couple of weeks, I was able to move into the Hope Lodge. The Lodge was located in a very tranquil wooded setting. It was operated by the American Cancer Society with support from Winn-Dixie Supermarkets. It housed 38 people in separate suites but has common areas that included the cooking and dining areas, library, computer and Internet facilities, laundry, and sitting areas.

When I checked into Hope Lodge I had quite an introduction to the manager, Jude Harrison. Once I was told that there was an available suite, I went by after treatment to scope it out. It was a suite overlooking the woods and it seemed to be ideal. I was excited. The next day I came to check in only to find that I was assigned to a different suite. Noting that the person at the front desk was different, and not knowing she was a manager, I immediately began to make a fuss. In a smiling and stern manner, I was told I could go back to my hotel! Well, Jude, I later learned, was once in the Marine Corps and she knew exactly how to handle all the men at Hope Lodge. We both began to laugh at this confrontation, and I quietly moved into my new suite, which I liked better.

While Jude tried to be a tough marine with us, she was actually a very sweet person, and often entertained us by playing the piano.

While I was there, 33 of the 38 residents were RCOG patients. This created a fertile environment for us to interact. Approximately half the men were accompanied by their wives who provided a nice touch to our Hope Lodge family. They became very much a part of many of the discussions we had about our experiences. The important role they played in helping their husbands face this disease was very evident. They were the same invaluable partner Juarez had been for me throughout my many trials.

Once my daily treatments became routine, the primary side effect was getting up three or four times each night to struggle to the bathroom half asleep. Overall, I was not suffering any fatigue from the treatment. This gave me more free time than I think I ever experienced during my adult life. I changed my treatment time from mid morning to the latest appointment time RCOG allowed at the end of the day. Then, my days were free for golf and other activities. At the lodge, we began to refer to our time there as our "radiation vacation."

I am a member of a national men's club, The Guardsmen, which has an Atlanta chapter. I spent a lot of time with my friends in this chapter who were very supportive and helped me immensely. With them and the men at RCOG, I played more golf than ever before and quickly realized that I had already peaked and my game would not improve enough for me to join the senior tour. This became an important social outlet for me while I was at RCOG.

 RCOG's treatment, and their overall program, was so thorough and non-intrusive that you could almost forget why you were there. However, every day that I went into the treatment room, meticulously aligned with laser beams that targeted tattoo markings placed on each of my sides and watched the radiation machine move over my body, I was reminded that I was in a fight for my life. If I won, I knew my treatment would end there, and if I lost, I knew it would mean the beginning of a lifetime of treatments. The other times that I came face to face with my true mission were the frequent trips to the bathroom throughout each night as I struggled with this physical impact of the daily radiation doses. I sent up many prayers throughout those nights as I was alone with just my thoughts and hopes.

As I got to know more of the men from other parts of the country who had made the journey to RCOG, it became apparent that an important aspect of our treatment extended beyond the clinic and involved our personal interactions and bonding. We ate together, spent a lot of time with each other and openly discussed our fears and hopes about prostate cancer. Once each week at Hope Lodge, we would have a potluck supper that would be brought in by an outside group, or we would prepare it ourselves. These were all social gatherings and this type of bonding turned out to be very important therapy.

At one of these gatherings, a fellow patient recounted how he had received a frantic call from RCOG the prior evening requesting he attend a meeting with the doctors first thing the following morning. He had a sleepless night. The next morning he arrived to find himself surrounded by a number of doctors all concerned about his health. He had completed the regular weekly questionnaire indicating some rather extreme side effects, but quickly explained that he may have exaggerated his condition. He was really OK. It appeared RCOG's doctors were, indeed, closely monitoring our condition via these questionnaires.

After listening to many of the men talk about their experiences facing prostate cancer, I felt their stories would be important to other men facing this killer. These stories could have greatly aided me in my search for a treatment. I decided to purchase a notebook and sit down with as many as I could to record their individual stories. So I began the process of interviewing and taking notes while I was going through treatment. This gave me something useful to do with all the time I had.

As each day passed and my treatment was drawing to a close I was frantically interviewing as many men as I could. I had initially anticipated talking with possibly five men, but the more stories I learned, the more interesting they became, and it seemed that each was different with its own unique message. When I finished, I had recorded the stories of twenty men! I didn't know how many I had talked with until I had compiled all of my data. Had I had more time, I would have gotten everyone's story.

I got to know some wonderful men and their individual Journeys of Hope. While we turned our weeks of treatment into a "radiation vacation," we never forgot the seriousness of our journey. We were battling the killer within to save our lives and the quality of our lives that we each cherished. Being together helped us wage our individual battles and the stories we shared made us realize that we were not alone: having someone to share with was important. However, our days together were drawing to a close as one by one we left to return home.

While the patients at RCOG and the men at Hope Lodge were from all parts of the United States and from other countries, I noted that very few were African American. While I was at Hope Lodge, there were four African Americans living there including myself. I attributed the low number to two factors: lack of widespread knowledge about RCOG and the high barriers associated with this treatment. These barriers include the treatment cost (many insurance companies would not pay for out of network, and/or out of state coverage), time away from the job, and the cost of housing, food, and transportation.

Many of us discussed these barriers, and since we bet our lives that RCOG had the best treatment available, we explored ideas on how RCOG could provide this treatment in other parts of the country. We raised this question at one of our seminar sessions and were told that the resources (trained doctors) to provide the treatments were not currently available and that RCOG didn't have any active plans to expand beyond the Atlanta area. In fact, while we were there, RCOG purchased two adjacent buildings and began the process of expanding into these added facilities. We remained hopeful that someday they would expand their service to other parts of the country.

On my last day at RCOG, I talked with Dr. Benton and went for my very last session with the radiation machine.

Alma Davis, a radiation treatment attendant, literally ran the treatment area and I had come to enjoy talking and joking with her daily. On this day, she presented me with my discharge instructions and we bid each other farewell. I walked through the clinic and said goodbye to the many other people I had come to know. Dr. Critz wanted to confirm I had received all the necessary discharge instructions. He took my package and went through it personally to double check. I thanked Dr. Critz, and said goodbye to him. He told me if I had any problems at all to contact him or Dr. Benton. While comforting, this was a stark reminder that I would be returning to Boston the very next day where I had no doctor to support my needs.

When I checked out of Hope Lodge, I realized I was also leaving my support group. But I would forever have the memories and the stories I recorded. These stories were in a spirit of sharing with each other, and each of us wanted to help other men understand and battle prostate cancer through our experiences.

The men I interviewed represent only a microcosm of the men diagnosed with prostate cancer each year. However, their stories will help to emphasize the state of affairs in the battle against prostate cancer and how men faced with this disease struggle in their approach to finding a treatment.

Their stories. . . .
(As told to the author)

Walter Bachmann, 67
Zurich, Switzerland
Business Executive

"Searching the World Over for the Right Treatment"

I began a new project in Czechoslovakia in 1990. I was hired as the CEO of the consortium of companies that led this project. As a part of the financing package, I was required to get a complete physical examination. Everything seemed to be fine according to the results. Some years later, I began to notice that I had problems with urination. I went to see a urologist for this problem in 1999. I had selected the best urologist in Switzerland, but because of the doctor's schedule, I could not see him until November of 1999.

In November 1999, I started a new project in Syria, responsible for developing and installing a new cotton mill and didn't keep my appointment with the urologist. The appointment was delayed until February 2000.

When I finally got my exam in February, I had an escalated PSA of 25. I had a biopsy the following day that showed prostate cancer, and a Gleason 7. The urologist recommended surgery with a treatment of hormones prior to surgery. He explained to me that the hormones were a form of chemical castration. I didn't want to lose my sexual potency. This was one of my major concerns with the treatment recommended by the urologist.

I began by researching the top prostate cancer centers in the United States and learning as much as I could. I learned of the side effects I could incur if I had surgery. I went back to my urologist to discuss treatment. The doctor was emphatic that surgery was my only choice, and disapproved of all other forms of treatment. With surgery as the only choice, I went back to Syria discouraged and continued my prostate cancer research.

I discovered that a friend in Switzerland, who was a medical doctor, was suffering from prostate cancer. I arranged a meeting with my friend who was near death. He told me he didn't trust surgery and had chosen external beam radiation treatment; however, prostate cancer had spread throughout his body and he eventually had the surgery. He also had taken hormone treatment, had an orchiectomy, and more radiation.

I was discouraged by my urologist's recommendation and after seeing my friend I was confused. I decided I didn't want to endure the fate of my friend, and seeing no other option, I decided to do nothing. I felt if I had to die from prostate cancer, it could be no worse than what I had witnessed with my friend who had undergone almost every treatment.

My family was strongly opposed to this "watchful waiting" course of action and urged me, with little success, to get treatment. I have a sister who lives in Chapel Hill, North Carolina and she knew a friend who had undergone treatment at RCOG. This friend was doing fine five years after treatment. My sister sent me information on RCOG's treatment.

I shared this information with my doctor friend who was suffering from prostate cancer. He referred me to a doctor within the University Oncology Department in Switzerland. The doctor was aware of RCOG and its treatment program and I asked for his opinion on treatment. He recommended RCOG's treatment over surgery.

I discovered that my medical insurance would not pay for it. I decided to pay for the treatment myself and sent my medical records to Atlanta. Dr. Williams telephoned me and said after reviewing my records, RCOG would accept me as a patient.

The doctors in Switzerland told me to be cautious about treatment in the United States. They said that the Americans were only business people and that RCOG's data was probably good because they only accepted the best patients in order to keep the data looking favorable. They also told me that the medical care in the United States wouldn't be good and I would be left on my own in the medical facilities. The doctors were not happy with me and felt I was running away to America while they had adequate prostate cancer treatment that was up to date. They believed I was "jumping into a spectacular treatment" that was untried.

I decided to come to the United States for RCOG's treatment in June 2000. My family was relieved and happy that I had decided to have treatment.

I feel the doctors in Switzerland left me absolutely on my own to research and find an appropriate treatment for my prostate cancer, and they were not supportive of my decision.

What I expected from RCOG's treatment has come true. The Hope Lodge experience has been fantastic. They are doing something good for people. American society is a great human-minded society and to live in America is a privilege.

I have decided to forget about the problems of prostate cancer and move on with my life. I know I will not be crippled by RCOG's treatment and will be going back home free of fear of physical restrictions. I must take care of other men who I know, because they aren't aware of prostate cancer treatment options. I am a member of a group of eleven men, all friends and co-workers, who were brought together in 1972 and trained to become industry and business leaders. Prostate cancer has been an issue with this group for a number of years. I now feel that I am able to advise them on this deadly disease.

Jack Bona, 70
Atlanta, Georgia
College Teacher and Opera News Writer

"Failed External Beam Radiation Treatment—Seeking Renewed Hope"

I had my first PSA test in 1992, while living in Florida. My PSA was 4, and my doctor told me that was an inconclusive reading and I should keep an eye on it. In 1995, I moved to Atlanta where I had another PSA test. The results this time were not good. My PSA was 5+, and a biopsy showed that I had prostate cancer with a Gleason score of 5.

When I was diagnosed, I was made aware of only two treatment options, surgery and external beam radiation. I chose radiation because I didn't want to go through the weeks of recuperation involved with surgery.

I had external beam radiation treatment in Atlanta during the month of June in 1995. Six months later, I became impotent. My wife had gone through breast cancer treatment right around the same time.

Following the radiation treatment, my PSA reached a nadir (lowest point) of 0.5 in November 1996. Afterwards, however, I watched my PSA steadily climb:

     March 1997   — PSA 0.7
     September 1997 — PSA 1.3
     March 1998   — PSA 2.2
     August 1998   — PSA 2.6

March 1999   — PSA 3.3
September 1999 — PSA 5.4

In October 1999, I had another biopsy that showed prostatitis, but not a recurrence of cancer. In March 2000, my PSA test was 5.8. This prompted another biopsy in May 2000, which showed a recurrence of cancer.

When I was originally diagnosed in 1995, I was told I had one shot for a cure. After being diagnosed a second time, I had mixed feelings about battling cancer again. The doctor's report was positive. They felt the cancer had not spread, but recurring cancer is recurring cancer.

I was never really depressed, even after all my years of battling cancer. In fact, I had begun to research various options after my PSA continued rising since 1997. After the cancer recurrence, I asked my urologist what the next step would be. My urologist had worked with Dr. Critz at RCOG and recommended that I contact him.

I have now completed my second prostate cancer treatment. I had no major side effects, and I feel positive.

Dr. Don Carlson, 67
East Molene, Illinois
Retired Dentist

"Looked for Bottom-Line Results"

I had been taking Saw Palmetto for four to five years, but I was having problems urinating. In April 2000, I was diagnosed with prostate cancer. I was not frightened when I was diagnosed and asked my urologist what would happen if I did nothing. I was told that I would probably live until my-mid 70's.

With my major concerns being quality of life and the side effects of treatment, I did extensive research on non-surgical treatments. I didn't consider surgery at all. People like to confide in their dentist and bartender. I had about 1,000 active patients before I retired and a lot of patients who had prostate surgery shared their stories with me. Every patient who had a radical prostatectomy with the exception of one, had incontinence problems, and most had become impotent. I had heard enough surgery horror stories.

In my research, I was impressed that Radiotherapy Clinics of Georgia was bold enough to publish the results of their treatment. I felt they must be producing results or they certainly would not dare to publish them in the current climate of medical suits and litigation. This gave me confidence in RCOG's treatment.

Being part of the medical community, I know that RCOG probably ticks off physicians and the prostate medical community because of publishing their results. I believe patients appreciate receiving data on RCOG treatment results and will hold them accountable. I am also of the strong opinion that not all doctors have equal abilities. When I was in medical school, half of the class finished in the lower half of the graduating class.

I feel that I will be cured. I considered not having any more PSA exams after this treatment, but to simply live my life and not worry any more about prostate cancer. However, because of the important research work being performed by RCOG, I plan to continue being tested and submitting the results to them.

I have seen six cases of oral cancer in my dental practice. The first three were cured, and the last three were not. This has shaped my life's philosophy. You do what you can the best you can and that's all you can do.

Albert Correia, 62
Danbury, Connecticut
Accountant

"Considered Living with Prostate Cancer"

In 1996, I had my annual physical examination. My PSA was measured at 4.0 and my doctor told me that if it went higher, I would need to see a urologist. When my PSA went to 6.0 in 1997, my doctor told me to get an examination by an urologist. I didn't go. In 1998 my PSA rose to 7, but I still wouldn't visit the urologist. Later in 1998, my PSA jumped to 8. At the urging of family and friends, I visited a urologist who gave me a biopsy that tested negative.

I had been doing some reading on prostate cancer and realized that things were not all good at this point. I went back to the doctor in September of 1999 and my PSA had risen to 9.5. I had another biopsy and it showed prostate cancer with a Gleason 6. During all these tests, the digital rectal examinations showed nothing.

The urologist wanted to immediately perform surgery. I refused. In December 1999, I chose a treatment course of natural homeopathic healing. This involved dieting, vitamin supplements, and exercise. I took all types of supplements.

My father had been diagnosed with prostate cancer around the age of 75. He lived to be 93 and died of something other than prostate cancer. I also had a cousin diagnosed at the age of 60 who lived to be 80. He had fifteen good years with no complications. The last five he suffered.

My PSA was taken again in January, 2000, and it continued to rise to 10. I decided to attend a support group in Danbury, CT, sponsored by the American Cancer Society, and found that people had chosen various treatments. I attended two meetings.

While I continued to administer my natural treatment, I lost 30 pounds, got in better shape and cured a lot of little illnesses; however, my PSA had risen to 11.2 by April 2000. My business partners started getting information off the Internet for me and I spoke with more people who had selected different treatment options.

I began to do some real soul-searching. I felt that if I did nothing, I might live to be 80, but if I took no action, my quality of life might not be worth living toward the end. I prayed and asked for a sign. In June, my PSA went to 13. I felt like this was the sign.

At one of the support group meetings, I met a gentleman who had completed RCOG treatment and was doing well, and I obtained RCOG information from him. I talked with my wife about RCOG and she concurred with a decision to have treatment in Atlanta.

In July 2000, I began my RCOG treatment. I had 152 seeds implanted. I feel very positive about RCOG's treatment. I think they killed the cancer.

James Driskell Jr., 52
Lakeland, Florida
Distribution Manager
Retail Grocery Company

"Guided By Prayer"

I started having PSA tests four years prior to my diagnosis. During the first two years, I felt all the tests were normal. In 1999, my PSA was tested at 3.6, and rose to 4.1 over a six-month period. I had a biopsy performed in November 1999, which was negative. However, within six months, my PSA had risen to 5.2, and my doctor gave me antibiotics to check any infections, then performed another biopsy. At this point, my PSA had risen to 5.9 and the biopsy showed prostate cancer with a Gleason 6.

When I was finally diagnosed, I felt empty, shocked, and confused even though my PSA had been steadily increasing. I had been getting up frequently at night to go to the bathroom, but I felt I was in good health.

I set up a consultation with my urologist two weeks after I was diagnosed. My wife, mother, father, and son all went with me to this consultation. We were afraid of what the doctor might say, but I knew from the beginning I didn't want surgery.

My urologist's first priority was surgery. My doctor also mentioned seed implants and radiation. I could sense that my doctor didn't understand what he was saying because he had mentioned earlier that seed implants weren't legal.

I left the doctor's office nervous and somewhat afraid, with lots of support from my family, but with a firm decision not to use this doctor if I did decide to have surgery. I went back home and prayed. At approximately 2 a.m. the next night, my wife and I got up and prayed again. We asked for guidance. I remembered a friend who had prostate surgery about four years earlier.

The next morning, I telephoned my friend to see how he was doing. He mentioned that his brother had been diagnosed with prostate cancer just eight months earlier and decided not to have surgery, but to have treatment in Georgia at Radiotherapy Clinics of Georgia. I met with my friend that evening and found him to be doing well after his surgery, but he recommended that I consider the treatment at RCOG.

After reviewing RCOG's information and visiting their clinic, I decided on their treatment.

I never consulted my urologist on my decision. Based upon my experience, I had no confidence in my urologist.

Otto Ewers,
Corpus Christie, TX
Business Owner

"Failed Cryosurgery—Still Hoping for a Cure"

I was first diagnosed with prostate cancer in March 1994 at the age of 54. I went to the doctor for my annual physical, and after my doctor performed a digital rectal exam he informed me that he didn't like what he had detected. Because of a low PSA reading of 2.2, I was not that concerned. However, my doctor referred me to a urologist for a biopsy—the results were positive.

I had a friend who was also diagnosed with prostate cancer, and had done extensive research on cryosurgery and other treatments. This friend was seeking alternative treatments to surgery because he was diabetic and had leukemia. He chose cryosurgery and had the treatment in February 1994. He seemed to be doing fine. With my wife, I decided to talk with the cryosurgery specialist. One of my primary concerns was whether cryosurgery treatment would eliminate the possibility of my getting another treatment later if it failed. The doctor told me that I would still have treatment options available. Based on this information, I decided to have the cryosurgery procedure at the John Sealey Medical Center in Galveston, Texas, even though I understood that I would be one of the first eight to ten patients receiving this treatment at that facility. The procedure was performed in April 1994, and I was back on my job three days later.

Cryosurgery seemed to be working for me. My PSA went down to 0.2. I had regular PSA tests after the treatment, but I was remiss in not logging my PSA test data to check my progression.

In April 2000, after an examination by my urologist and with a PSA of 2.2 I was diagnosed with prostate cancer for a second time. I had experienced no symptoms prior to the first or second diagnosis.

Being diagnosed with prostate cancer again, was the second biggest shock of my life. My biggest concern now was whether cancer had spread to other parts of my body. My fear was heightened by the fact that I lost a dear friend to prostate cancer in January 2000, after unsuccessful surgery.

With this new diagnosis, my urologist said he would schedule radiation treatment immediately. I told my urologist I had rushed into a treatment decision before, and this time I intended to do a thorough analysis of my options. My urologist didn't agree with my position.

While I was visiting a friend in Seattle, he told me about a procedure there that I should evaluate. My friend telephoned the Seattle Center for me. The doctor at this center mentioned the treatment provided by Radiotherapy Clinics of Georgia and actually forwarded a brochure.

I turned my focus to RCOG in an effort to determine if I was a candidate for their treatment, after having been treated by cryosurgery. After telephone calls and eventually forwarding a letter to Dr. Critz, I found out four weeks later that I could be treated by RCOG. My treatment was scheduled to begin July 27, 2000.

I have now completed my second prostate cancer treatment. If I had access to the same information in

April 1994 as now, I would not have chosen cryosurgery. I feel great about RCOG's treatment and believe I have been cured. However, my friend who had cryosurgery in February 1994 is still doing well, with no signs of recurrence and a PSA less than 0.1.

Randy Friday, 47
Birmingham, Alabama
Mortgage Loan Officer

"Youth is No Barrier"

I began having regular PSA tests six years ago at the age of 41. I was paranoid and felt I had prostate cancer even though no one in my family had it. My PSA tested high and my doctor gave me antibiotics. I requested a biopsy but my doctor saw no need for it at that age. In April 2000, I had my very first biopsy and was diagnosed with prostate cancer. My PSA was 4.8 with a Gleason 5.

I had a lump in my throat when I was diagnosed. My associate pastor was diagnosed with prostate cancer in his late 40's or early 50's and he was dead in less than two years.

I also recalled a friend who was diagnosed with the same PSA reading as mine. My friend had surgery and the cancer came back in five years. He then had radiation treatment, but the cancer returned four years later. Now he is taking hormone supplements. From this first-hand experience with prostate cancer, I figured I wasn't going to die soon. I'd probably have up to ten years to live.

My urologist outlined my treatment options as radiation seed implants, or surgery. He told me that he could do the surgery, and gave me a booklet to read. Surgery seemed a difficult procedure to master. This scared me even more. When I asked the urologist about cure rates, he told me that he didn't keep up with them. At this point, I began doing research on the Internet and found RCOG. My wife and I visited RCOG in May 2000 and were most impressed with their treatment program.

I never talked to my original urologist again. I did, however, get a second opinion from another urologist at a university hospital. This urologist advised me, whatever I did, not to go to Atlanta (RCOG). He didn't give a reason.

I began my RCOG treatment in June 2000. I didn't like having to go to Atlanta for two months, but I was very pleased with the treatment and I enjoyed being with the other men at Hope Lodge.

My original urologist sent me a letter in September 2000 telling me it was time to reschedule my appointment. He doesn't know that I have completed my treatment.

Dan Graham, 51
Milwaukee, Wisconsin
Business Executive

"Battling a Family History of Cancer"

I lost both my father and mother to cancer and I recognized that I probably would have to deal with cancer at some point in my life. I started inquiring about my PSA at the age of 45, even though my doctor had told me I didn't need to be concerned about my PSA until I reached 50.

As soon as I turned 50, I had my PSA checked. When I was 51, my PSA tested at 4. I was told to come back in six months. In six months, my PSA had risen to 7, and my doctor immediately referred me to a urologist for a biopsy. When my urologist telephoned me with a message that I had a small amount of cancer, I accepted this with a sense of resignation. The hardest part was telling my wife and two sons.

My urologist discussed treatment options with me and told me about surgery. I immediately dismissed it because of the side effects. My wife, Cindy, and I then explored other treatment options. We studied external beam radiation and seed implants. We also discovered RCOG on the Internet and were encouraged by the information and data that RCOG presented.

Cindy and I visited RCOG and we were impressed by what we saw of the clinic and by our discussions with the patients there. We consulted RCOG doctors and were able to get our questions answered. We also visited Hope Lodge.

Over dinner, while still in Atlanta, Cindy and I made the decision to have treatment performed at RCOG. I began my treatment in July 2000. I feel very good about this treatment option as opposed to surgery. I also feel optimistic that if this is the extent of the cancer I have to deal with in my life, then this treatment has cured it.

Charles Gray, 51
Pensacola, Florida
Freight Train Conductor
Combat Veteran

"Blames Agent Orange"

In 1999, I had a PSA that measured 4. My doctor told me that it was normal. In February 2000, I had another PSA test that had risen to 8.7. After a biopsy was performed, I was told that I had prostate cancer with a Gleason score of 5.

My urologist wanted to immediately perform surgery. However, my wife, Emma, was busy doing research over the Internet to find other treatment options.

I was a member of the 101st Airborne Division and served in Vietnam in 1967 and 1968, during the Tet Offensive. As an infantry rifleman, I was part of a seven-man team that would be dropped into the jungle to set up ambushes—in the middle of Agent Orange spraying.

My father is 78, and I have brothers who are 58, 55, and 48. Within my immediate family, I am the only one who has ever been diagnosed with prostate cancer. I believe my prostate cancer is directly related to my combat activity and Agent Orange. I have seen a lot of veterans diagnosed with this disease. President Clinton signed a bill for veteran benefits that cited Agent Orange as a contributing factor to prostate cancer.

I didn't consider the Veterans Hospital for treatment because of what I had seen of other veterans treated there for prostate cancer. Prostate cancer is a primary topic of conversation among veterans.

I considered surgery but didn't like the potential side effects or the thought of not being cured by this radical treatment. I also considered brachytherapy and took two hormone shots while I was considering treatment options.

Emma's Internet research led me to RCOG. After discussions with RCOG doctors, I decided that this was the treatment for me.

I completed RCOG's treatment with no side effects. My outlook is positive and I believe my cancer is gone. The seminars at RCOG have been very helpful, and I know, now, how to handle prostate cancer. I believe people should start having PSA tests as early as possible—in their 40's.

Author's note:
According to Chapter 1, 38CFR paragraph 3.311b
Presumption of Exposure;

A veteran who served in the Republic of Vietnam during the Vietnam war shall be presumed to have been exposed to ionizing radiation. (note, this extension was signed into law in June 1998) Veterans who are diagnosed with prostate cancer should contact their local Veterans Administration representative. Service connected disability may be possible.

Jack Kaufman, 71
Boise, Idaho
Navy Commander, Retired
Professor Emeritus

"Precious Friends"

I never had any prostate problems during my lifetime, though in 1994, I did have kidney stones. During treatment for this, my urologist gave me a PSA test. I know now that my PSA was 5.2 at that time, but my urologist never told me this. In 1996, at my 50th high school reunion, I vividly recall a classmate, who lives in Atlanta, giving me a brochure and suggesting I read it. This classmate said to keep it handy because if I lived long enough I would have prostate cancer. I read it and threw it away.

In September 1999, my PSA tested at 5.8. I reviewed my records for the prior six to seven years and found out that my PSA had always been high. A biopsy showed prostate cancer with a Gleason 6. I was absolutely devastated, and told my wife, Shirley, that the most frightening thing that could happen to me was to hear the "C" word. My urologist told me that he would do surgery.

One of my friends, a fellow church member, had chosen surgery and I set up a lunch meeting to get his guidance. He told me that if he had it to do again, he would not do surgery. He handed me the same brochure that my classmate gave me some years prior. This firend's uncle had been diagnosed the same time as he had, and begged him to go to RCOG. He had refused and now the fellow church member was incontinent and impotent from his surgery.

I immediately contacted RCOG and went down for a visit. I spoke with patients and RCOG doctors. My doctor told me that I was absolutely crazy to go to Atlanta for RCOG's treatment. He told me that the best procedure was to remove the prostate, get radiation or seed implants, but not to do both. I was convinced my urologist was not up to date on current treatments. I decided on RCOG's treatment and brought a brochure to my urologist. His assistant assured me that he would not read it. I have had no contact with my urologist since I made the decision on RCOG's treatment.

Me and my church member friend are considering starting a prostate consultation service for the men in our church.

Peter McGrath, 57
Birchwood, Tennessee
Chemical Engineer

"Analyzed Treatment Options Prior to Cancer Diagnosis"

I began having annual PSA tests in 1992. In 1996, my PSA had exceeded 4.0, which I considered a dangerous threshold. I had a biopsy performed, but it proved negative. At this stage, I started researching information and data on prostate cancer and treatment options, in an effort to be prepared.

After extensive analysis I made the decision in 1998 to have treatment at Radiotherapy Clinics of Georgia, if I were ever tested positive.

From 1996 through 1999, my PSA was tested at 4.0, 7.0 and 11.0. All biopsies still proved negative. In the Spring of 2000, my PSA rose to 15. I decided to go to Vanderbilt University Hospital for a different testing venue. This biopsy, which was my fourth, showed prostate cancer.

The notification of cancer was expected, and I was not disturbed. In fact, I slept soundly.

I telephoned RCOG and told them that I wanted to come there for treatment and be completed by September 15. My urologist talked to me about surgery, but I had spent years researching and studying treatment options. My choice of treatment was firm. I met with RCOG doctors and told them that I was "pumped up and ready to go that day."

With a PSA of 15 and a Gleason score of 8, I was informed that I would require lymph node dissection as a part of my treatment.

I began my treatment the morning of July 17, 2000. After I was admitted, the doctors came in with a new Gleason reading of 7. With this downgrade, the lymph node dissection was cancelled as I lay on the operating table. My surgical treatment was limited to RCOG's standard seed implant and conformal beam procedure.

I have not lost any sleep over having prostate cancer. I think I selected the best treatment option and now feel that the cure is in God's hands. The key for my positive outlook was knowing the treatment options and understanding there is a cure.

Collins Munns, 59
San Diego, CA
Retired Mental Health Director

"Selected Watchful Waiting for a Magic Bullet Cure"

In the early 1990's, I insisted on a PSA test even though my primary care physician had reservations about the need for one. My PSA was normal. I continued to get PSA tests annually. In early 1995, I received a PSA reading of 4+ and I was referred to a urologist who told me that African Americans had a higher incidence of prostate cancer, and recommended a biopsy. In November of 1995, I was diagnosed with prostate cancer, with a PSA of 6+ and a Gleason 5.

I had stopped eating red meat in 1975 and turned to a "healthy diet" that included nutritional foods along with supplements. I had also undergone hip replacement surgery in 1994. The diagnosis of prostate cancer was a shock, and the thought of having this disease brought on a sense of anger and frustration along with immense fear.

My urologist was very cautious in discussing cancer with me. He outlined all my options for treatment, but made no specific recommendations about any treatment. I later found out that my urologist had been shot by an outraged prostate cancer patient when he became impotent after surgery.

I began a journey of research to better understand prostate cancer treatment options. I went back to my urologist to discuss the results of my research to find that the doctor was not well versed in the various forms of treatment. I then transferred to the head of urology of my insurance carrier and established a relationship with him who promoted cryosurgery as a treatment. I also consulted an independent urologist.

My insurance carrier recommended surgery or external beam radiation. I explored my options thoroughly over a three-to-four- month period starting in November 1995. I didn't like the side effects caused by surgery, nor did I like the odds. My urologist was urging me to make a decision quickly.

I made a conscious decision to pursue the "watchful waiting" option at the age of 55, against the advice of each of the urologists I was consulting.

Beginning in 1996, after I made this decision, I began attending prostate cancer conferences and began a journey in search of the "magic bullet" cure. I wanted to be the first in line for this miracle treatment when it became available. I continued to monitor my PSA, which stayed "relatively low." I also increased my dedication to a strict dietary routine that included soy products. However, I decided not to use Saw Palmetto or any other substance that might "artificially" lower my PSA.

In early 1999, my PSA rose to 10 and I became concerned. Toward the end of 1999, my PSA had risen to 15. I became a little frantic and realized that watchful waiting was not working and the "magic bullet" cure had not been found.

My new research led me to discover RCOG. While my urologists were skeptical of this treatment, they recognized RCOG's research and peer- reviewed publications as being valid. I made the decision to get treatment at RCOG in March 2000. At that time my PSA had risen to 21.4. Because of this high level, I also had to have lymph node dissection.

I would like to have known about RCOG five years earlier, but I think I have taken my best shot. One thing that bothers me most about prostate cancer is that it is a silent killer. I have never had a symptom since I was first diagnosed.

Gordon Albert Pritchard, 59
Feilding, New Zealand
Owner, Specialty Wood Products Firm

"Faced with Long Odds"

The government in New Zealand discourages doctors from doing PSA testing. However, when I went to my doctor in mid-March 2000 for a physical exam, I asked about nutritional supplements for the prostate. My father had prostate problems and I wanted to take precautions. My doctor asked if I wanted a PSA test. Later, I called the doctor's office to ask about the results of my general physical. I also offhandedly inquired about the results of my PSA test. The doctor's nurse told me that it was "OK." I then asked what my PSA reading was, and she told me 37! On visiting my doctor again, he referred me to a urologist.

The urologist performed a biopsy and found that I had cancer in all six needle samples. I was told by the urologist that I didn't "need" surgery. While surgery is the recognized top treatment in New Zealand, my cancer was considered too advanced for it.

Tests to determine the spread of cancer all proved negative. The urologist gave me a prescription for hormone treatment. I saw a radiation specialist who advised against radiation, telling me that it would not prolong my life, but only fry my insides, and make me impotent. Another urologist had recommended an orchiectomy. This process of consulting various specialists took three months.

When I was told I had cancer, I wasn't freaked out, but I wondered where the doctors were coming from with their advice.

My best treatment option in New Zealand seemed to be hormone treatment. However, I had begun researching treatment options over the Internet and found RCOG. On the advice of RCOG doctors, I had a lymph node dissection performed in New Zealand. This procedure showed only a trace of cancer in one node, though, during this period, my PSA rose to 46 with a Gleason 8.

RCOG accepted me into its treatment program, which began in July 2000. I feel good about this treatment. I hope for a complete cure. If not, I expect to get some additional years—whatever I get is a bonus.

I have faced cancer before. I lost my first wife to breast cancer when our two sons, now ages 33 and 31, were just teenagers. I am prepared for the battle with prostate cancer.

Don Radcliff, 53
Business Consultant
Atlanta, Georgia

"Balanced Cancer Treatment with Fathering a Child"

In 1997, I had an examination for allergies. In performing a range of blood tests, my doctor discovered that my PSA was 4.2. This doctor referred me to a urologist who performed a biopsy that was negative. The urologist recommended massive doses of vitamins and surveillance of my PSA. In February 2000, I requested a PSA test, which showed a rise to 6.2. A biopsy showed that I had prostate cancer. A bone scan and MRI test for spread of cancer proved negative but it was recommended that I get cancer treatment by the end of the summer.

My wife, Pamela, went with me to the urologist's office to get the results of the biopsy with the intent of tape-recording the treatment options and recommendations, but the doctor wouldn't let us. During this meeting, we asked the doctor about seed implants and were told they didn't work well. The urologist recommended surgery. I asked about alternative treatment options and was told that none of them worked very well. I told the doctor that I would seek a second opinion.

I never talked with my urologist after that visit, nor did I ever hear from him. I began to explore the various treatment options without the guidance of a doctor. I found RCOG on the Internet and was convinced this was the best treatment option. I met with RCOG doctor,

Hamilton Williams, who told me they could provide treatment.

During the initial consultation, I informed Dr. Williams that Pam and I were interested in having a baby. The doctor referred me to another urologist. I had had a vasectomy 17 years earlier. Pam and I had an appointment to go to Houston, Texas, to have a reverse vasectomy when I was diagnosed with prostate cancer.

Dr. Williams of RCOG located a doctor in Atlanta to handle the vasectomy reversal. He had a different procedure that I now think is superior to the one in Houston.

The first procedure performed by Dr. Williams was to extract sperm from me with needles and implant them in Pamela's egg, but it didn't work. This procedure was performed in May of 2000. Another procedure, where a testicle was opened under local anesthesia, was performed at the end of June.

I was getting somewhat anxious about starting prostate cancer treatments during these procedures. A procedure could only be performed once a month, if the second procedure failed, it would be July before we could try again. The second procedure worked! I called RCOG immediately to scheduled PC treatment and my treatment began at the end of July.

Because of the radioactive seeds implanted by RCOG's treatment, Pam and I could not be together during her pregnancy. We used separate bedrooms and couldn't get any closer than 4 to 6 feet of each other, until around the end of December 2000. All tests showed our baby to be healthy and the birth was expected in March 2001.

During this entire course of events, the only disturbing time for me was the day before the seed implant at

RCOG. I didn't know what to expect. I feel that I was always able to balance the needs of conceiving a baby with PC treatment. Im upbeat and positive, and expect to be cured of prostate cancer.

Don and Pam Radcliff became the parents of a healthy baby girl, Richlyn, on March 23, 2001. An important part of his overall treatment is now successful!

Charlie Reynolds, 63
Ft. Walton Beach, FL
Retired Engineer

"Used a Support Group to Evaluate Treatments"

I began tracking my PSA when it was less than 1.0 because I had seen the devastation of prostate cancer when a close friend was diagnosed in 1990 and died in 1997. My friend had undergone surgery, radiation, chemotherapy, and an orchiectomy in his battle.

In 1999, my PSA rose to 4.2 and it was creeping up by about 0.2 ng/ml every six months. In March 2000, my PSA had risen to 4.6. I had a biopsy and was diagnosed with prostate cancer.

I had a six-needle biopsy that left me with a serious infection. This prevented me from being able to schedule a CAT scan and MRI for at least six weeks. Unable to determine whether the prostate cancer had been contained, or spread to other parts of my body, I endured a prolonged period of anxiety. However, I did start attending a prostate cancer support group in April.

The support group consisted of approximately thirty men and it was sponsored by the American Cancer Society. The support group provided me with the best information that I received from all my research. Within this group I was able to interact with men who had received all types of treatments. The group had gathered literature and information from many treatment centers around the country. Also, at times, doctors attended meetings to discuss various treatments. From this experience, I felt I had been exposed to all treatments available for prostrate cancer.

The support group leader had received radiation treatment that had failed. He found that hormone treatments were high maintenance and very expensive, and it was necessary to take other medications to counteract its side effects. Some men were on PC-SPES and other dietary programs, but they were not able to determine if they had any effects. I saw where the high dose rate (HDR) treatment left a patient with a high PSA in bad shape.

I completely ruled out surgery while attending the support group meetings. I observed that almost without exception, men who had undergone a radical prostatectomy, suffered from urinary incontinence, and some had received surgery more than five years earlier.

During these meetings, my fear and anxiety mounted as I was awaiting the opportunity for further testing so I could decide upon my treatment options. During this wait I also observed two men who had undergone treatment at RCOG. I noted that one had no problems after he had been treated five years prior and the other, ten years prior.

Based upon my new found knowledge, I reasoned that with a PSA of 4.6 and a Gleason 7, cancer cells had probably penetrated outside the prostate gland and the treatment I received should address this condition. I chose radiation.

The only treatment center I found that performed seed implants, followed by external beam radiation, was RCOG. I talked with the two members that had been treated at RCOG, reviewed their cure rates and decided this was my best option.

When I started treatment, I felt positive because I had done a complete analysis of my treatment options and felt the treatment I chose offered me the best hope to maintain my quality of life and be cured.

I found the Hope Lodge a great experience! I was able to interact with other prostate cancer patients in a supportive atmosphere. I am looking ahead to a declining PSA and being cured of this cancer. I have a very positive outlook for the future.

Kenneth Scott, 63
Lawton, Oklahoma
Farmer

"About Ready to Cash Life In"

I began following my PSA in 1996. I saw a urologist who told me that my prostate was a little enlarged, but he hadn't felt anything on the digital rectal exam. Even with a PSA of 7.8 in 1998, he didn't give me a biopsy. I hadn't studied the appropriate PSA levels and I didn't realize how elevated they were.

In 1999, I went to Scott-White Clinic in Temple, Texas, for an examination. When I returned home, I had a message waiting from them, indicating that my PSA was high and I needed to immediately see a urologist and get a biopsy. I saw a different urologist who found prostate cancer with only a two needle biopsy.

The urologist informed me that the cancer was aggressive, PSA 11.7 and Gleason 8. He wanted to give me a hormone shot to slow it down. I scheduled a another appointment at Scott-White Clinic for a second opinion.

I had suffered from severe medical problems and I was devastated by the prostate cancer diagnosis. I was just recovering from these other medical problems, now cancer. I was about ready to cash it in. I had enough with being sick.

I talked with a number of people who had prostate cancer surgery and I was not prepared to go through this process. My daughter researched alternative treatments for me and found RCOG on the Internet. We were impressed with the data available on the ProstRcision treatment, and the non-surgical nature of it.

I talked with doctors at RCOG and with two people in Oklahoma who had experienced RCOG treatment. These men highly recommended the treatment and had experienced no side effects three years later. Based upon these discussions and the data available from RCOG, I elected RCOG for my treatment.

I began treatment at RCOG in June 2000. The treatment presented me with no side effects other than a little fatigue. I believe that if my cancer is cured, I'll be in good shape.

RCOG is well organized, but they are getting crowded as more people find out about their treatment.

William (Bill) Seidel, 70
Titusville, Florida
Retired Engineer

"A Long Road"

My prostate problems began in the late 1980's when I was diagnosed with an enlarged prostate. I was given medication to help alleviate the problem, and later during this same period I had a TURP procedure. My doctor told me there were suspicious "spots" on my prostate, but with a PSA less than 4, not to worry. Another urologist gave me the same opinion. My PSA started to rise each year and I had biopsies performed in 1996 and 1997.

After I was scheduled for a second biopsy in 1997, a series of unusual events took place. The biopsy was to be performed while I was under general anesthesia. This required me to see my primary doctor to get verification that my physical condition was OK. My doctor performed a complete physical examination including blood work. When the doctor received the blood work report, he thought it was wrong and had me give another blood sample on a Saturday morning. Later that same morning, the doctor rushed to my home in a state of complete alarm. He had discovered that my blood platelet count was just 5,000. A normal count is 140,000. I was immediately hospitalized for this condition and the biopsy was postponed. This ordeal lasted a full six months before I recovered.

After recovery, a new date was set for the biopsy. Again, I went to my doctor to get the clearance required for hospital admission. A new doctor examined me and requested an EKG. The EKG revealed an abnormal heart condition. He gave me a thalium stress test. The result was a blockage in my heart. I was again hospitalized, this time for further tests and treatment. Two stents were inserted into one of my arteries.

I was able to finally have a biopsy performed in July of 1999, and while vacationing in August 1999, I was informed that I had prostate cancer. Being an ordained deacon in my church, I attributed my ability to survive this ordeal to my faith in God.

I went back home in November 1999 to face the cancer. I discussed treatment options with my urologist. My PSA was 7.4 with a Gleason score of 6.

My urologist was against surgery and suggested seed implant or watchful waiting. I decided upon the seed implant (brachytherapy) treatment. To shrink my prostate for the seed implant, the urologist began an initial program of hormone therapy, which was to continue for a period of up to nine months.

While on this phase of my treatment, I discussed my situation with one of my friends who had the same stage prostate cancer, and was being treated by the same urologist. My friend had been doing research over the Internet to explore other treatment options. This friend discovered RCOG and passed the information on to me.

I reviewed all of RCOG's information, statistics, and data on cure rates. I spoke with RCOG's Dr. Williams and decided that this was my best treatment option. In February 2000, I stopped my hormone treatment and prepared for RCOG.

I like the treatment here and believe I made the right decision and will be cured.

After this treatment, I plan to go back to my cabin in the mountains and finish my vacation.

Willard Snyder, 64
Bank CEO
New Tripoli, Pennsylvania

"Chose a Path of Dieting and Prayer"

I was first diagnosed with prostate problems in 1985 when tests revealed that I had an enlarged prostate. In 1990, my PSA was 5. At this point, my doctor put me on notice to watch my PSA. In 1997, with a PSA of 8, I had my first biopsy, and it was negative. However, with a PSA of 8.3 in 1999, I had another biopsy in November and was informed on Christmas Eve that I had prostate cancer.

A strong faith in God is a central part of my life and I went through the Christmas holidays with lots of prayer. My plan was to beat prostate cancer through dieting and prayer. I changed my diet to fruits, vegetables, and fish, and I saw a chiropractor who administered herbal medications. I followed this program for three months.

In March 2000, I had another PSA test, which showed that my PSA had climbed to 11. At this point, I decided to do prostate cancer research using the Internet. I also went back to my urologist who recommended that I have surgery. The urologist let me know that I would probably become impotent as a result. Though this factor disturbed me, I went ahead and scheduled surgery.

I had discovered RCOG while doing my Internet research. My wife, Lucille, and I decided to go to Atlanta, Georgia, to attend one of RCOG's Tuesday night meetings. During this trip, I met with RCOG doctors and discussed my situation. On my way home, I decided RCOG's treatment was my best option. I called my urologist on my cellular phone and cancelled surgery. I scheduled my RCOG treatment to begin at the end of June 2000.

The lowest point during my ordeal was when my PSA rose to 11 after my dietary and herbal care effort. I now feel very positive about the prospect of being cured. My pastor told me that maybe I was led to RCOG for treatment so that I could spread the word to others. This has brightened my outlook.

Robert Stewart, 64
St. Claire Shores, Michigan
Photographer

"Guided by His Wife with Divine Intervention"

I had my first PSA test in February 2000. It read 25. I was diagnosed with prostate cancer in mid-March with a Gleason score of 7.

I felt that the problem would be fixed and I was not overly concerned. I knew very little about prostate cancer, or the function of the prostate gland.

Surgery was ruled out as a treatment option because of my high PSA. I had limited my options to radiation or hormone therapy. I talked with a radiologist about treatment and working this treatment around my schedule as I traveled and continued my photography business.

My wife, Mary, had a much more serious perspective of prostate cancer. She researched information on the Internet to gain an understanding of treatments.

While Mary was doing her research, I had decided on radiation and was scheduled to begin external beam radiation treatment on the Friday following Memorial Day, June 2, 2000. On Sunday, May 28, 2000, Mary told our Pastor about my health problem and my treatment plan. The priest held me by my shoulders and told me he hoped the Holy Spirit would guide me in making the right decision.

The next morning, Mary turned on her computer, typed in "Radiation Therapy" and Radiotherapy Clinics of Georgia appeared on the computer screen. Mary interpreted this as a message from God, in response to the priest's call for guidance from the Holy Spirit.

Mary gave me all the data she had gathered off the computer with a cover letter from her. In this letter, she told me she knew we were not communicating and she wanted me to take my health problem more seriously. The next day, while in the shower, it finally came to me: I had a bigger problem. I also realized that I was lost and didn't know what to do. Mary immediately called Radiotherapy Clinics of Georgia. RCOG suggested not starting radiation treatments until I spoke with their doctors. An RCOG doctor telephoned me that evening. The next day, I cancelled my external beam radiation treatments.

I met with RCOG doctors on July 3 and had a lymph node dissection on July 5, along with the seed implant. The lymph node dissection proved negative.

I have a positive outlook on this experience, and I look forward to a complete cure. In addition, as a high-profile individual in my community, I plan to let people know my story in hopes of increasing prostate cancer awareness and imparting a better understanding of the treatment options available to men diagnosed with this disease.

Chapter IX
A Journey Of Hope

Ten years is a long time—it is a decade—120 months—520 weeks—3,650 days. However you choose to measure ten years, it is a long time, and the standard measure used to define disease freedom from prostate cancer after treatment. This is the journey of hope that I, and the other men with me at RCOG, must travel successfully to be considered cured. By my estimation we will join approximately 1.5 million other prostate cancer survivors on this journey.

The ten-year standards for disease freedom (cure) for the radical prostatectomy (RP) and ProstRcision treatments are identical—0.2 ng/ml PSA readings or lower. However, they are approached from opposite directions. For RP, the 0.2 PSA nadir should be reached within six weeks following treatment. After reaching this level men are regularly tested for up to ten years to make sure the PSA does not rise. If it rises above the 0.2 level, this is a sign of cancer recurrence and treatment failure.

Prior to our treatment completion at RCOG, we received a seminar on what to expect with our PSA post-treatment readings. Our PSA levels are expected to fall over a period of time to the 0.2 level and remain at this level or lower as we continue our regular PSA tests over a ten-year period. RCOG provided a table of what to expect with our PSA levels over time based on pre-treatment PSA levels. This table is presented here. The PSA reading for each month after treatment (3-42) represents the median PSA for each PSA group.

To illustrate a median PSA, if the PSA of 101 men was measured at 12 months dated from implant, the median PSA would be the PSA of the 51st man. Thus, 50 men would have a PSA falling faster than the 51st man and 50 men would have a PSA falling slower than the 51st man. RCOG points out that it is very important to know that it does not make any difference how quickly your PSA falls. According to their data, where cure rates have been calculated for men with fast- falling PSAs and slow-falling PSAs, RCOG has found the resulting cure rates to be identical for fast- and slow-falling PSAs.

PSA Group Before ProstRcision

Follow up Mos	0-4.0 ng/ml	4.1-10.0 ng/ml	10.1-20.0 ng/ml	>20.0 ng/ml
3	1.2 ng/ml	1.8 ng/ml	2.6 ng/ml	3.7 ng/ml
6	0.8 ng/ml	1.1 ng/ml	1.6 ng/ml	2.0 ng/ml
12	0.5 ng/ml	0.6 ng/ml	0.8 ng/ml	0.9 ng/ml
18	0.4 ng/ml	0.5 ng/ml	0.7 ng/ml	0.6 ng/ml
24	0.4 ng/ml	0.3 ng/ml	0.5 ng/ml	0.5 ng/ml
30	0.2 ng/ml	0.2 ng/ml	0.2 ng/ml	0.4 ng/ml
36	0.1 ng/ml	0.1 ng/ml	0.1 ng/ml	0.2 ng/ml
42	<0.1 ng/ml	<0.1 ng/ml	<0.1 ng/ml	<0.1 ng/ml

If we don't have any cancer recurrence (as determined by the post-treatment PSA), then our battle with prostate cancer is behind us. If cancer recurs, then we have a lifetime battle ahead of us. And this journey becomes a never ending, tough Journey of Hope—based on today's technology.

Each of us chose RCOG and their ProstRcision treatment because we believed it offered us the very best chance for a complete cure. RCOG's overall seven-year cure rate with this "new" procedure is 89% (94% for my PSA group). RCOG projects the ten-year cure rate to be no lower than 85%. We all are hoping and praying to be in this number.

My pre-treatment PSA group is (4.1 – 10.0). My three month post-treatment PSA was 1.0, the six-month follow-up PSA was 0.6. On July 11, 2001, I was tested for my twelve-month follow-up. My PSA was 0.4! This compared very favorably to the twelve-month median PSA of 0.6. My PSA levels, at this time, were falling faster than the median! Since I was never on hormone treatment I know that these PSA readings are valid and not artificially lowered. While I am pleased with these results, I know that they are very preliminary and I am on a long Journey of Hope. If my PSA falls to 0.2 and stays at this level or below for the accepted ten-year cure point, then I will celebrate cancer freedom. This battle, which began with my trip to Atlanta on July 4, 2000, will then become my personal holiday. I have faith that I will celebrate my independence from prostate cancer. However, for now, I will celebrate each milestone that I successfully reach, as my PSA is tested every six months.

Overall, my health journey began when I met that special stranger—my angel at the West Concord Donut Shop. After two years on this journey, I am a very blessed man.

My blood sugar level remains normal and I have never needed to take diabetes medication since I first stopped the medication in June 1999. I have remained on the Atkins diet "maintenance" program. This allows me to eat well, maintain my weight, and successfully handle my former diabetes problems. This component of my overall health has been the most noticeable for me.

As part of our follow-up information to RCOG when we send our PSA test results, we complete questionnaires to keep RCOG appraised of our sexual function, and any urinary or rectal side effects. After receiving the maximum dose of RCOG's conformal beam radiation treatment, I had some concerns in these areas. However, I have suffered no urinary or rectal problems. My sexual function is normal without the aid of any stimulants (Viagra or others). Considering that I had accepted losing my normal sexual functions through the surgical treatment, this is certainly a major benefit of ProstRcision.

I have remained in communication with the other men who were with me in Atlanta. The PSA test results show that we are all on the road to being cured. Everyone I have spoken with, aside from one reported no lingering side effects from the treatment.

As each man who spent the summer of year 2000 in Atlanta continues his personal pursuit of cancer freedom, we are filled with renewed hopes. We hope that the flawed prostate medical care system will be overhauled and improved so that other men won't have to struggle as we did to find their best treatment. We hope that medical science will continue to make breakthroughs in its research on the prevention, treatment, and elimination of prostate cancer. And most importantly, we hope to help end the killing silence surrounding prostate cancer that is impeding all progress.

We accept that ending the silence will need to take on many forms in order to be successful, but men individually can begin this process immediately. We all can start by bringing up the subject of PSA testing to family, friends, and associates on a continual basis, making this a topic of discussion as natural as talking about the weather. At some point, those who do not have a good handle on their PSA will get the message. Men can ask their primary care doctor what he or she knows about prostate cancer and their views on PSA testing. If it is clear the doctor doesn't know enough, find another doctor. If your PSA is rising, take Peter McGrath's approach and begin analyzing the various treatment options, and select one where there is a comfort level before being faced with a cancer diagnosis.

Once referred to a urologist or oncologist, immediately ask them for their treatment cure-rate data for both five- and ten-year periods, and be sure they state these facts in measurement terms that are fully understandable. If they do not have this historical data, find someone else. Like any other business, the doctors will get the message if they do not get the business. If diagnosed with prostate cancer, don't panic. Talk with as many men as possible who have gone through treatment and learn from their experiences. Always obtain multiple opinions on your condition and don't be forced into a hasty decision. All of these are steps that each man can take today. I believe the entire medical system needs to evolve into a much more responsive system. It will when we force it to do so.

One and a half million men traveling a Journey of Hope is a large number of combatants in the prostate cancer battle.

What should I do along the way? That is the question that I ask myself as I begin my journey. I am sure others must ask themselves the same question. Then, I imagine if we all became active—what a thunderous sound would be heard from this raging battle as we traveled together along this journey. This would propel prostate cancer into its rightful place in the public consciousness and help generate the resources we need for widespread education, awareness, and research, and to overhaul the medical care system. On this very day, approximately 100 men in the United States alone will die from prostate cancer—most of them in silence. While watching television and seeing the accounts of approximately 75 men, women, and children who die from automobile accidents a day, imagine the benefits of giving our journey that level of visibility. And, since prostate cancer is curable, we must ask ourselves how many of these 100 men could be saved.

Prostate cancer has already claimed three of the men I loved most in this world and it threatens both my sons, as they, like me, are in high-risk groups. I have to believe that for all the 1.5 million men traveling this Journey of Hope, one of everyone's strongest desires is that our sons and grandsons either avoid or be cured of this disease.

When I first saw the men in RCOG's lobby awaiting treatment, unafraid, I knew that these men, like me, were ready for battle. As I came to know them in our day to day treatment for prostate cancer, we became a team, a brotherhood, supporting each other as we battled this killer. Prior to going to RCOG, I spoke with a number of men who were very helpful to me. Some of these men I only spoke with over the telephone and I do not know whether they were white or black, millionaires or penniless, PhDs or high school dropouts, but they each reached out and offered support as members of the team. All of these men have been a blessing to me.

There are prostate cancer survivors volunteering across this country working in support groups and other organizations who are reaching out to men all along this journey, and making an enormous impact. From their actions, these men are at war with prostate cancer, and they are my heroes. Charles Austin, a Boston television news reporter, is an inspirational example. Diagnosed in 1995 at the age of 50 with a PSA of 650, a Gleason grade 9, and metastasized prostate cancer, Charles is a six-year survivor with a PSA that is now 0.2. Not only has he defied all odds, with a strong faith in God and prayer, coupled with near miraculous medical treatments that are continuing, but Charles is one of the most active prostate cancer advocates within Massachusetts. When he heard of my diagnosis he called to offer his support.

I will always remember Bill and Margaret Frisbee for their work and support while I was in treatment at RCOG. Bill Frisbee is a minister who was diagnosed with prostate cancer and obtained treatment at RCOG. After his treatment he had a first hand appreciation of the fear and agony that men go through, so he dedicated his ministry to this battle.. Each month, as men and their wives came to Atlanta for treatment, the Frisbees' invited them into their home for an evening of sharing, food, and general socializing. He also hosted a weekly prayer breakfast.

However, to maximize and amplify on these heroic individual efforts, I believe we must somehow focus this brotherhood of survivors to openly declare a war on this killer within. What would we seek to accomplish with a declared war on prostate cancer? I would include among our objectives those cited below in bold:

Widespread Education and Awareness, Especially for Those at Highest Risk

This must be our first objective because it is vital to achieving every other victory. Also it is an area that we can, to some extent, impact directly because the men at highest risk are our family members, sons, brothers, nephews, uncles, etc. How many times have we seen brothers and other family members battling prostate cancer at the same time? I have seen it often. After I completed my treatment at RCOG, I learned that my father's youngest brother, who is one year younger than me, had been diagnosed with prostate cancer. Within a span of twelve months, my father died from prostate cancer, I was diagnosed and treated, and his brother was diagnosed. This killer is relentless within high risk groups. Now that we know about prostate cancer, we need to bring together our friends and family, educate them, and recruit them into our war. In addition, we must demand and force public sponsored education for all men.

When I was told I had prostate cancer and realized I knew absolutely nothing about it, I was embarrassed. I kept asking myself, how could I be so dumb? I saw this lack of knowledge as a personal failing.

I tried to learn everything I could as quickly as possible, but this was no time to be introduced to my prostate. The shock of cancer was not conducive to learning. Later during treatment, when I began to talk with the men in treatment with me, I realized that my lack of knowledge was the norm and not the exception. Is this lack of knowledge a reason that men keep prostate cancer closeted? Not knowing how to communicate with the urologist and other doctors on the subject surely could cause most men to follow the doctor's advice without questions and make them less likely to talk openly about their experiences. Can they feel comfortable with their knowledge? I know that the men in my family have been violated by prostate cancer and I also know that we have been totally dysfunctional relative to battling this killer. Unfortunately, we are a typical family.

Education also needs to begin before we are diagnosed, even before our PSA begins rising. According to certain studies, our diets can be linked to prostate cancer. The nutritional program at RCOG focused on eating certain foods and avoiding others. For all men, and again, especially those at high risk, this knowledge is needed much earlier in life when it might have its biggest impact in actually preventing the disease.

It is absolutely necessary for us to have basic knowledge of the prostate as we enter adulthood? How can we protect ourselves if we are introduced to our prostate gland when it becomes cancerous?

I didn't miss the prostate lessons. That information didn't fail to reach me. The necessary educational outreach does not exist and it must be a centerpiece in our war.

Standardization, Physician Training and Accountability

The flawed prostate care system based on my experience and as seen through the stories of the men with me at RCOG, is fairly easy to understand. It is based upon the business principal of providing treatment services to a defined set of consumers. Each doctor providing a service views the men afflicted with prostate cancer as business accounts. The problem that we must tackle with our war is to learn to act like the consumers that we are. Prostate cancer treatments constitute a multi-billion dollar industry. This means that each year, men are spending these dollars out of our pockets, or directing our insurance carriers where to send these dollars.

I am very comfortable with this business arrangement because it should allow us to maximize our strengths since there is no monopoly involved. In the classic business-consumer relationship, the consumer dictates the quality and level of service by choosing where they shop and from whom they purchase. After understanding the prostate treatment business principles, I, along with the men whose stories you read, went shopping and chose RCOG to provide us with their treatment services.

RCOG provided a level of detail about their service that we could understand and use as a basis for making our decision. The overriding problem within the prostate cancer treatment industry is that most service providers do not provide adequate information. We must force them to change their practice or go out of business for lack of accounts. This is standard business practice. Why should we allow it to be different when our lives are at stake?

Under the present system, some doctors are not current in their knowledge, this has again been demonstrated through all of our stories. Why should they be rewarded with our business if other doctors are investing in training, and keeping their practice current, and providing details on their practice results.

Our actions can, and should, force all the service providers to outline their training, experience, cure-rate history and the standards used to measure results. Once this information is available, then all men can choose where to buy their service. These actions will then force a better overall quality of service as the service providers who want our business become better and stronger while offering an increased level of service. The service providers who are getting along today without making an investment in their business will surely fade away. I believe that the better service providers will applaud the actions we take in this area.

Public Visibility and Support

"Cancer is a political, as well as a medical, social, psychological and economic issue. Every day, government policymakers make decisions that affect the lives of more than eight million cancer survivors, their families, and all potential cancer patients."

The American Cancer Society Annual Report, 1999.

This is a powerful statement highlighting one of our major weaknesses, which should actually be one of our key strengths. The silence surrounding prostate cancer has greatly minimized it as a political issue and positioned the number one cancer afflicting men as almost politically impotent. However, with an army of 1.5 million, plus recruits, we can quickly change this scenario.

I have had a great deal of experience advocating for policymaking support at all levels of government, and it is my sense that our elected officials, at every level, would support and join in a war on prostate cancer. What elected official would not support a goal of awareness, education, and outreach to men, or would not support a call for better treatment services. Our war on prostate cancer must outline and present our needs and recommended solutions to elected officials in a way that allows them to respond with the support we need.

We must also make the general public aware of our plight through public outreach campaigns. Elected officials will react to the agitation of their constituents, and that includes the general public as well as ourselves.

Politically, the number one cancer among men must rise to the forefront so that the decisions made will impact positively on our families and all other potential prostate cancer patients. The National Prostate Cancer Coalition (NPCC) appears to have taken a leadership role in promoting political action. The NPCC Web site can be found at www.pcacoalition.org.

Adequate Resources

I do not know the amount of public or private money invested each year in prostate cancer programs. I have confidence that it is not equitable relative to the amount invested in the fight against other diseases of comparable devastation. I believe this is a fact because my experience tells me that silence is rarely rewarded, especially in an environment such as ours where the battle for resources is highly competitive. Our war has to be aimed at successfully competing for and obtaining our fair share of resources. While we, many times, blame the doctors (and rightfully so, at times) we have left them at a distinct disadvantage in not demanding more resources to support their efforts and other medical initiatives.

One area where adequate resources are needed is for research and analysis. Why can't standards be established around PSA testing? Are there other issues causing such divergent positions on something as fundamental as PSA testing? What research needs to be performed to give uniform guidance to the public?

When we look at adequate resources, we need to have a full appreciation for the overall resources allocated to prostate cancer for fighting cancer and other high-priority diseases. I would expect that prostate cancer needs advocates, that is our role as part of our war on prostate cancer.

Eliminate the African American Disparity

Why is the incidence and mortality rates among African Americans so much higher than others in the United States? Why was it almost certain that with my family history and being African American I was destined to face prostate cancer? Why are my sons, and all African American sons, at the highest risk? Are African Americans doing something detrimental to our health or are we suffering this higher affliction rate because of a genetic makeup? What are the problems causing such a disparity? While I have seen and studied the very depressing statistics, I do not see the answers to these questions. Who is focusing their efforts on answering these critical questions and what resources are being allocated to their efforts?

Imagine if all Americans suffered the incidence and mortality rates faced by African Americans, then we would be looking at an overall incidence approaching 300,000 annually and approximately 100,000 men dying from prostate cancer each year. These would be panic conditions attracting broad attention and the necessary resources to find some answers. This is the real life situation among African Americans now, but where is the panic? Where is the priority and most importantly, where are the resources needed to understand and address this health crisis?

Our war on prostate cancer must focus on this disparity as a high-priority objective. Surely there must be some answers explaining this disparity and once they are known, there must be some actions that can be taken to reduce or eliminate a disparity of this proportion. Immediately there must be some accountability to African American communities that regularly report on the efforts now underway and the preliminary findings. In addition, until some significant progress is made, resources should be provided to station "prostate care specialists" in these high risk communities.

A Cure for Prostate Cancer

Why not make this our bottom line objective? Recall Collins Munns in search of a "Magic Bullet Cure." Can our actions help facilitate and expedite efforts in this area? Certainly!

With more educational and awareness initiatives, increased political power and public visibility, and more resources, we can position our focus on finding the "Magic Bullet Cure." There are research initiatives currently underway to find this cure. Some of this research is focused on gene therapy, and I am sure there must be other initiatives. But have you heard or read anything on these efforts? The research on prostate cancer, again, the number one cancer among men, is as silent and hushed as the men suffering from this disease. We must have public visibility and accountability in this area.

With God's blessing and power, we can win this war on prostate cancer. My story began when God sent me a messenger and I continually called upon God for guidance throughout my darkest hours. Robert Stewart, James Driskell, Jack Kaufman, and William Snyder, in all their stories, cite the power of prayer and God's blessing.

One of the blessings that we have witnessed throughout most all our stories is the presence and support of our wives and loved ones—a support that is woven all along this precarious journey, without which many of us would be without hope at this very moment. It was my wife who forced me to get an exam, which eventually led to the detection of cancer and put me on this journey. Look at the stories of the men with me at RCOG and how their wives supported them. I saw this support firsthand as many of the wives stayed with these men throughout their treatment. Surely, they will join us in our war on this killer, as they, too, want to protect their sons and grandsons.

As we travel along this journey, some of us will be cured, some will successfully battle this killer throughout their lives and others will be taken away from this world by prostate cancer. Like my father and grandfathers, I may be in that number that is taken away. If I am, I want to leave not having traveled a silent Journey of Hope, but as a casualty of war where victory is won. Knowing that my sons, and grandsons—not yet born—will beat this killer. I have to believe that every man on this journey shares this goal.

A Journey of Hope Prayer

O God, you have taught me from my youth, and till the present I proclaim your wondrous deeds,

And now that I am old and grayheaded, O God, forsake me not

Till I proclaim your strength to every generation that is to come.

Your power and your justice, O God reach to Heaven,

You have done great things; O God, who is like you?

Though you have made me feel many bitter afflictions, you will again revive me;
from the depths of the earth you will once more raise me.

Renew your benefits toward me, and comfort me over and over.

So will I give you thanks with music on the lyre, for your faithfulness, O my God!

I will sing your praises with the harp, O Holy One of Israel!

My lips shall shout for joy as I sing your praises;

My soul also, which you have redeemed, and my
tongue day by day
shall discourse on your justice;

How shamed and how disgraced are those who sought
to harm me!

Amen.

Psalm 71
Verses 17 through 24

Chapter X
Winning

On April 18, 2005, I celebrate the five-year anniversary of the beginning of my battle with prostate cancer. It has been a celebration because prostate cancer has not adversely impacted my life. Since I completed my treatment at the Radiotherapy Clinics of Georgia (RCOG) in the year 2000, I have not needed any medication or further treatment; most importantly, I have not suffered any side effects.

When I reflect back so vividly on the day that I received the telephone call from the urologist informing me I had prostate cancer and when I recall the overwhelming fear that had, at the time, consumed me, it seems like a lifetime ago. In many ways, it was another life. Through my personal encounter with prostate cancer, I have become passionate about addressing the needs of other men who are at high risk of stumbling into a battle with this "killer within" and being as unprepared as I was initially. The work that I do in this area has changed my life and my overall perspective. It has presented me with an opportunity to have a positive impact on others. When men who have read *Battling the Killer Within*, or who have attended one of my workshops, tell me that I saved their lives, it is truly a uniquely rewarding experience. This experience gives me the impetus to press forward with the war on prostate cancer, and guides me as I travel my personal journey of hope.

The first chapter of this book, entitled "Sweet Victory," recounts my experience of better understanding diabetes and taking actions that I thought could help me beat the disease. When I originally wrote about this experience in the year 2000, I had successfully come off my diabetes medication. Today, five years later, I have never needed to go back on any medication. I continue better eating habits and all tests now indicate that my diabetes is completely controlled. My experience with diabetes is significant because it was my first in taking control of my health, which gave me the confidence to face prostate cancer.

My personal experiences with prostate cancer and diabetes are important examples of winning strategies that can help other men. After five years of talking about prostate cancer with others, I am convinced that the prerequisite to winning is to conquer fear—to first win the psychological battle. Conquering fear does not mean eliminating it; this may be impossible. What it means, instead, is relegating fear to the background and not letting it drive your decisions. Most men do not like to admit they are frightened, but it is a normal emotion when facing a killer. Naturally, I still have an underlying fear of the disease that took the lives of my father and grandfathers. Conquering fear is going to be a most difficult challenge for some men, and may necessitate some form of counseling. Some men use psychological and, or, spiritual counseling. Don't hesitate to seek out and use the services needed to effectively stabilize and push fear and depression to the background. This will not be a strike against your manhood, rather part of your winning strategy.

Conquering the fear of prostate cancer is truly a tremendous challenge. The best advice is to prepare yourself to face this disease during your lifetime. A proactive approach is especially important for those men who are at high risk for the disease. Through education, awareness, and discarding outdated inhibitions, you are preparing to conquer fear and, ultimately, win the psychological battle.

Education and awareness, as I have said, play a primary role in your battle plan. Understanding how the prostate works and how to monitor its health is the first step. The health of your prostate can largely impact your sexual health. This realization alone should give some added importance and priority to monitoring your prostate health. In this era of widespread advertising for sexual enhancement or erectile dysfunction drugs such as Viagra, Cialis, and Levitra, you should not be embarrassed about openly discussing your prostate health and its impact on your sexual health. The prostate is a precious sex organ; without prostate health, sexual dysfunction can become an issue, and the drugs mentioned above could become useless. My doctor made it perfectly clear to me that my surgery would lead to impotence.

Men, especially those at high risk for prostate cancer, should not wait until they are diagnosed with cancer to be introduced to their prostate. For men at high risk, winning a battle with prostate cancer should start early in life.

By the age of 30, talk with your doctor about prostate health. Even though it is rare for a man under the age of 35 to develop prostate cancer, I have seen such cases. Learning how to talk with your doctor about the prostate also goes a long way in overcoming a major obstacle in prostate health—the culture of silence surrounding the issue. So, protect yourself, learn where the prostate is located, how it functions, and symptoms of prostate disease. There are resources listed in this book that can guide you during this discussion path, (see appendices 1 and 4).

As you are introduced to your prostate, you will invariably learn about a healthy diet and nutritional supplements that are intended to help maintain your prostate health. While I offer no advice on whether any of these are helpful, certain dieting and supplements have been tested and offer anecdotal evidence of success. My advice is to discuss these options with your doctor; if you are at high risk for prostate cancer, I suggest you arrange a counseling session with a urologist or oncologist, as well as a nutritionist.

Once you get to know your prostate, the next step is to learn your family history, and your prostate cancer risk level. Remember, no one is exempt from developing prostate cancer at some point in their lives, regardless of family history. But taking the time to talk with family members and gather information can help you assess your risk. If you cannot obtain the information needed, then perhaps a cautious approach is to assume that you are at high risk, "high-risk plus" for African American men.

All men with a close family member (grandfather, father, brother, or uncle) having been diagnosed with prostate cancer are considered at high risk for this disease. For African- American men meeting these conditions, the risk is even higher, putting them in the category of high-risk plus, due to an incidence rate that is the highest in the world.

The mortality rate disparity for black men in the United States is 140 percent greater than any other race in the United States. This means that African-American men die at a rate 2.4 times greater than other men. This is the largest racial mortality disparity for any cancer afflicting men or women.

There are many factors contributing to this disparity. For African-American men, cancer tends to strike at an earlier age and is detected at a later stage than for other men; education and support is obviously an absolute must in closing this disparity.

Another factor that puts you in a high-risk category is exposure to the chemical Agent Orange. This chemical was widely used in the Vietnam War. For a case history, review the story of Charles Gray and his experience on page 119 of this book.

Family history, race, age, and possible chemical exposure are all considered risk factors for prostate cancer. Armed with knowledge about your prostate and your family history, the next step is to monitor your prostate.

Monitoring your prostate health is done through PSA blood tests and through digital rectal examinations. These are the universally accepted "screening" procedures. The age recommended for you to begin monitoring your prostate depends on your risk level.

It is generally recommended that men who are not deemed high risk should begin screening at age 50. Men at high risk should begin at 45, and some recommend that men designated as high-risk plus should begin at age 40.

Knowing that prostate cancer can be cured with early detection, I personally believe that a critical aspect of beating the disease is monitoring prostate health through screenings.

I know men at the highest risk level who do not get screened because they fear knowing whether they have cancer. I certainly understand this fear, but the fact remains, monitoring your prostate health early on is essential to winning. I know other men who will not have a digital rectal exam (DRE) performed as part of their annual screening, saying that it "violates" their manhood. (Many times, prostate cancer is detected through a DRE when the PSA tests "normal.") Well, recall the story of

Otto Ewers, (see page 112) and think what's more violating—a DRE or an autopsy?

Fear comes from feeling vulnerable. If you are at high-risk, you must arm yourself with knowledge, regular screenings, and awareness.

Even five years after my diagnosis, the debates within medical circles surrounding screenings rage on. In fact, if anything, these debates have become more intense. In 2004 we have witnessed major news stories emanating from research indicating that – (1) Using the PSA standard of "4" as an indicator of a prostate problem is too high and should be lowered; (2) The PSA velocity should be used as the key indicator of prostate health regardless of what the PSA level may be; (3) Men are being treated unnecessarily for prostate cancers that may not harm them; and, (4) The usual argument that PSA testing has not been proven inconclusively to save lives. In essence, it seems that there has been no significant change from the debate status quo over the past five years. The bottom line is that men have to make decisions about monitoring their prostate health and cannot become frozen in place until these debate issues are resolved.

These sometimes conflicting facts drive the current medical debates, but men and their families have to educate themselves and learn to sort through these facts to make informed decisions about their health. In preparing to beat prostate cancer, it is important to track the results of your screenings. Often, men will tell me that they have been screened and that their doctors say they're fine. When I ask them what their PSA reading was, they have no idea. I can't emphasize enough the importance of becoming involved in the management of your prostate health. Knowing your PSA readings and tracking their change from year to year means taking responsibility for your health and being proactive in the protection of it. Meet with your doctor after each screening to review your results, compare the new results with the prior year(s), and note the changes. If your PSA is rising from year to year, note how fast it is rising. This is known as the PSA velocity and could indicate that you have a prostate problem regardless of what your PSA levels are. If you are being screened annually at a free screening center, be sure to obtain the written results of each screening and maintain these records so you can compare and discuss the numbers with your doctor. Appendix 19, a "Personal Prostate Health Management Guide," is provided to assist you in understanding your risk level and assembling and monitoring your PSA and other test data. The guide will provide visibility into the condition of your prostate health.

If your PSA is rising at a seemingly high velocity, you must treat this very seriously. In other cases, some men with rising and/or elevated PSAs are biopsied without any signs of cancer being detected. My message to both groups is to "plan on facing prostate cancer and plan on beating it." If there are signs that a problem could be on the horizon but you have not yet been diagnosed, then a good strategy is to begin preparing your battle plan. A number of helpful steps can be taken in the event you are diagnosed at a later time. Go back and review the story of Peter McGrath (Page 123) to see, firsthand, how this strategy worked for him.

Some specific steps that I recommend when facing danger signs are

1. Begin researching your treatment options and obtain a good understanding of each treatment.
2. Research treatment centers and their history of success in treating prostate cancer.
3. Visit support groups, find one that you are comfortable with, and attend meetings; prostate

cancer survivors are the very best source of information for items 1 and 2 listed above.
4. Talk openly with your immediate family about the danger signs and prepare them for your possible battle; get them involved in your preparations.

When you take these steps in the face of danger, you are already winning half the battle. Getting in the frontlines of this battle psychologically will prepare you for the physical part of the battle, should it be necessary. Think of the time invested prior to a cancer diagnosis as an investment in education, or an insurance policy. There are times when you are called upon to use your education and there are aspects of an education that are never used. We hope this education will never be used, but that it is available to you should you need it.

Taking a proactive approach by getting to know your prostate, getting screened, and preparing yourself psychologically will drastically reduce fear and uncertainty in the event you are diagnosed with cancer. You will have also placed yourself in the position of facing prostate cancer on terms favorable to you; early detection and a proper treatment plan is the best combination for a complete cure. The time and effort put into this approach could very well be the deciding factor in winning a battle against prostate cancer.

* * *

I would expect that many men reading this book will do so after being diagnosed with prostate cancer. This is precisely where I began my personal prostate cancer battle. My message to you is that while the initial terms of battle may not be the most favorable, you still can win!

If you are facing prostate cancer unprepared, you are probably struggling mightily with fear and just beginning the psychological battle. Having been there, I understand what you are going through. The very fact that you are reading and searching for answers means that you have not buried your head in fear and anguish. This is a very positive first step.

The fear of cancer seems to be a universal fear, and it is almost certain that your family is shocked and in fear as well. You are probably seeing a lot of concerned faces, some tears, and hearing soft words of encouragement from others. This type of caring and concern is to be expected and appreciated. However, you must quickly move beyond this initial stage of your encounter with prostate cancer because you have to prepare for what may very well be the fight of your life. You should identify those around you who will be positive and supportive and who can help you prepare a plan to beat prostate cancer. After you have assembled your team of family members, doctors, and friends, I suggest that you avoid discussions about your condition with curiosity seekers. You and your team will need all of your time and energy to focus on developing a winning plan.

There was a time when I believed the only way to beat prostate cancer was through a complete cure. This is no longer my view. If a man is able to manage this disease and maintain a good quality of life, then he is winning the battle. Your perspective on this battle is important because a number of men will be diagnosed with conditions that may seem almost impossible to beat at first glance. However, I urge you not to give up. Regardless of your condition, you still have a chance to beat prostate cancer.

I want to again bring to your attention my good friend, Charles Austin. As I pointed out five years ago, Charles was diagnosed in 1995 at the age of 50 with a PSA of

650, a Gleason grade 9, and metastasized prostate cancer. The doctors gave Charles little hope of surviving, but he did, and did so with a remarkable zest for life. In 2004, Charles was an announcer at baseball games for World Series Champions the Boston Red Sox. In addition, he continued his very active and outstanding efforts to help educate and support other men. Charles has never given up, and his example shows that a winning attitude does matter!

When faced with prostate cancer unprepared, men become vulnerable to a needless rush to treatment. A proper approach still has to be put together based, once again, on solid knowledge and a clear understanding of your options. Your urologist or oncologist may want to rush you quickly into a treatment. Remember, it is likely that by the time you are diagnosed, you probably had prostate cancer some months or years before even being diagnosed. A rush to treatment may not be a wise approach. Do not let fear drive your decisions and cause you to make a misjudgment that may cost you your life or your quality of life. If Charles Austin could conquer fear and make the right decisions at his stage, then so can you.

Your options after a prostate cancer diagnosis are treatments, or watchful waiting. If you decide to have treatment, then you must decide which treatment is best for you. Unless you have meticulously monitored your prostate health and prepared to face and beat prostate cancer, these are decisions that will now require time and study. These decisions should be made with the team you have assembled. Appendix 11 provides summary information on various treatments including watchful waiting—use it as a guide to begin an in-depth analysis of your treatment options. Once I made my treatment decision, I sealed it with a prayer. I believe I have been blessed through prayer, and I recommend it.

Older men, I believe, have to be very cautious in approaching prostate cancer treatment. Two important facts surrounding prostate cancer again come into play. Some men live with prostate cancer untreated and without suffering and, prostate cancer treatments can have damaging side effects. When considering these facts for older men, the right choice can become complicated.

Often, for older men, children and grandchildren are the ones leading the research and driving the decision-making process. So it is important for them to understand that prostate cancer may or may not harm their loved one during his lifetime. I suggest a thorough review of the prostate health screening history and the overall health of the loved one. Consultations with a urologist, oncologist, and primary care doctor are important in helping to assess the overall health of the loved one. Clearly understand the benefits and risks of the various treatment options beginning with the least invasive. Also understand the benefits and risks of watchful waiting. Multiple opinions may very well be in order in deciding whether to treat or not, as well as the best treatment option if treatment is selected. Quality of life issues should be a major factor in your decisions.

Men and their families will select treatments for prostate cancer whether they have prepared a plan before diagnosis, or after diagnosis. At whatever point preparations begin, most men enter treatment hoping and praying for a cure. The ultimate goal is a complete cure with absolutely no side effects. Some men achieve this goal through their initial treatments. Each year, countless prostate cancer survivors enter the ranks of cured survivors. These men have been blessed and rewarded for their treatment preparations and good decisions. For these men, their battle with prostate cancer ended in victory.

CR Thomas A Farrington

The battle against prostate cancer for some men, however, will continue after their initial treatment. I can imagine that facing prostate cancer again after completing a treatment must bring back the original fear, or an even greater fear. Whether you have just completed a radical prostatectomy and have been told that cancer has escaped the prostate gland and is still present, or you find your PSA rising again years after your initial treatment, your winning attitude must continue. Focus on conquering your fear and moving forward with another battle plan for prostate cancer and again plan on beating it.

Manny Hammelburg, a friend in the war against prostate cancer, who lives in the Greater Boston area, has an interesting story of perseverance and a winning approach. Manny was diagnosed with prostate cancer in 1987 at the age of 47. This was before the use of PSA screening, so he didn't know the exact details of his condition. Manny's father had been diagnosed with prostate cancer, so he was at high risk for the disease. Manny had external beam radiation treatment in 1987. He had his first PSA test in 1989, which was hovering around 1.0. Over the years, his PSA would eventually rise to 6.8, which signaled that his encounter with prostate cancer was not over. In fact, his 1992 tests determined that prostate cancer had metastasized to his spine and hip. Manny chose and underwent an experimental chemotherapy program at the National Institute of Health in 1992. This treatment caused renal failure and his doctors did not think he was going to survive. He did, however, and since 1992 his PSA has tested negligible (0.05). Manny was on hormone treatments for seven years, but stopped taking this treatment in 1999. In 2005, Manny is an eighteen-year prostate cancer survivor who is very active within the Massachusetts Prostate Cancer Coalition and other organizations within Greater Boston, helping educate men about facing prostate cancer.

Whenever I see and talk with survivors, I urge all these men to become active in the war against prostate cancer. Not only is this an avenue to help others, but it is also a way to stay current with new developments in treating the disease. Too many survivors tend to distance themselves from the overall war after their treatment. I believe factors driving this disassociation may include not wanting to be identified as a prostate cancer survivor, trying to put a frightening experience behind you, or not understanding the significant contributions you can make. This disassociation, in my opinion, is not prudent on two fronts. First, your experience and involvement could help other men; and second, your disassociation prevents you from learning and staying abreast of new treatments that you may eventually need yourself.

I have seen many men pronounce themselves cured of prostate cancer immediately after surgery when the urologist tells them that tests show no further spread of the disease. My prayers and hopes are with these men that their cure is complete and no further treatments are necessary, and this will be true for many men. However, the standards for a complete cure are a negligible PSA ten years after treatment. As much as we pray and hope that we are completely cured after our initial treatments, we cannot be sure for many years.

What I have realized since my treatment ended is that my active involvement with helping others puts me in constant contact with leading prostate cancer medical specialists and researchers. I am continuously learning about new developments, and if I have to battle prostate cancer again, I know whom to talk with and what new treatment technologies are available. A prostate cancer survivor's active participation in the war against prostate cancer is helping to beat prostate cancer in the global sense. More education and awareness, more research, more public visibility and support are all issues that will gain momentum with increased participation from survivors. This war must be led by the prostate cancer survivors themselves, along with their families.

Stan Klein, another survivor and friend in the Greater Boston area is a model of what can be done through a personal commitment. Stan was diagnosed with prostate cancer in 1993 at the age of 64 with a PSA of 69 and a Gleason grade 9. He chose surgery (radical prostate-ctomy) as his treatment. Following surgery, his doctor confronted him with the news that his margins tested positive and he still had prostate cancer within his body. Four months later, Stan began an external beam radiation treatment that lasted seven weeks and ended in March 1994. Doctors told Stan's wife, Fran, that the prognosis for a cure wasn't good. Stan is now an eleven-year prostate cancer survivor whose PSA was undetectable in October 2004.

Stan started attending a newly formed prostate cancer support group in 1994 at the Deaconess Hospital in Boston, Massachusetts. This group expanded to other Boston hospitals and assumed the name of the Longwood Medical Area Prostate Cancer Support Group. Stan is now the facilitator of this support group.

In September of 2000, the American Cancer Society awarded Stan with the Sandra C. Labaree Volunteer Value Award because of his work with the support group. Stan realized that prostate cancer did not have the visibility and support within Boston that it deserved. Stan says that as he looked out on the audience at the John F. Kennedy Library upon receiving his award he announced, "Next year, there will be a walk for prostate cancer within Boston." This was the first time he told anyone of his idea about this new effort. Fran said she was "shocked" at his announcement and tried to "slide under her table." Afterward, Dr. Jeffrey Steinberg (a noted urologist affiliated with the Beth Israel Deaconess

Medical Center in Boston, Massachusetts), joined this nascent effort as cochair.

Beginning every year since 2001, the Boston Prostate Cancer Walk is held on Father's Day on the Boston Common. Through 2004, the walk has raised funds and awarded $540,000 to Massachusetts' medical institutions to support prostate cancer research. The amount in 2004 represented seventy percent of the funding for "new" prostate cancer research initiatives at Massachusetts' medical institutions, according to Stan. The walk also funded an educational videotape that has been distributed to more than one hundred communities within Massachusetts, Rhode Island, and New Hampshire. The walk that Stan envisioned in 2000 began with 1,400 participants in 2001 and attracted 5,000 participants in 2004. Fran has committed herself to Stan's vision and her work is a major contribution each year to the success of the walk. The Boston Prostate Cancer Walk is one effort toward winning the war on prostate cancer. The work it supports will help save the lives of men as they wage their personal battles against this killer.

Winning the battle against prostate cancer has to be understood and accepted on a personal and universal basis. These goals are inseparable, as much as some men may want to consider their personal battle as an isolated case independent from everyone else. The personal battle is a journey of hope that will span a number of years. The work of the likes of Charles Austin, Manny Hammelburg, Stan Klein, and others will be a personal life saver for many men in years to come. All survivors should remember their sons and grandsons are also at high risk or high risk plus, so your work in this battle can help find a cure for a close family member. There is enough room for all prostate cancer survivors to use their experience and talents in the war against this disease, and they are needed.

Since my treatment, my personal battle with prostate cancer has consisted of a PSA test every six months. While I have suffered no side effects from my treatment, I did experience a PSA bounce. A PSA bounce is a phenomenon associated with radiation treatment where the PSA suddenly increases after treatment and, just as suddenly, falls back down. Radiotherapy Clinics of Georgia doctors had made me aware that there was a possibility I would experience this bounce. This bounce caused me to talk with my doctors at RCOG on several occasions to get some assurance of what I was experiencing. So far, and thankfully, I have been able to turn my attention from my personal battle to the universal war on prostate cancer.

In 2003, I founded the Prostate Health Education Network, Inc., (PHEN). PHEN is a 501(c)(3) nonprofit organization focusing on the education and awareness needs of black men in the United States—the men with the highest prostate cancer incidence and mortality rates in the world. PHEN is focused on helping to eliminate this vast disparity by targeting key factors contributing to it including lack of knowledge concerning risk levels and screening guidelines, access to screening, and involvement in prostate cancer support groups.

In 2004, PHEN created a model program in Boston that will be replicated in other cities. This program began with PHEN recruiting a cadre of black prostate cancer survivors who meet monthly to develop strategies and plans and work on PHEN projects. PHEN developed working partnerships with leading medical and cancer centers. The Dana-Farber Cancer Institute became PHEN's primary partner. Working with more than thirty community groups including churches, health centers, barber shops, retail businesses, and the Boston Transit System, PHEN placed prostate cancer education and awareness posters around the city. With support from the Radio One Boston affiliates, (WILD and WBOT) and the

Bay State Banner newspaper, PHEN is able to distribute information via public service announcements. In collaboration with Dana-Farber Cancer Institute, PHEN has established Boston's first prostate cancer support group targeting black men. Working with the Dana-Farber Cancer Institute and community health centers, PHEN is now establishing ongoing education and awareness workshops coupled with free screenings. PHEN has also established a Web portal for online education and awareness and for providing information on prostate health and cancer resources for twenty-five U.S. cities with large African-American populations. (www.ProstateHealthEd.org) The support of my family has been a critical factor in the early success of PHEN. My wife, Juarez, brings an unparalleled level of energy and creativity to PHEN initiatives. Tomeeka, my daughter, who now owns a public-relations firm, keeps the organization visible through the various media outlets within Boston and nationwide. My son Trevor lends support to our programs, and Chris, my oldest son, is ready to jump into action when PHEN begins its activities in his city of New York.

When I reflect on what PHEN has accomplished, I am pleased with the initial progress. I am most proud of the prostate cancer survivors who have dedicated their time and talents, and each and every one has made, and continues to make, significant contributions. This is the model that will have to be repeated within cities across the country to help eliminate the African-American disparity. I am excited about the prospects of accomplishing this goal—a challenge that will certainly not be easy. All prostate cancer survivors should realize that addressing the world's most egregious disparity will support the overall war on the disease, and subsequently their family members as well.

For most men, battling prostate cancer will begin as a very personal battle filled with hope and fear. Once you conquer the fear and concentrate on preparing a plan and winning this battle, amazing and sometimes miraculous results are possible. You realize that you can beat prostate cancer, even if it takes more than one battle to rid your body of the disease. When you travel your personal journey of hope, you are presented with the opportunity of using your experiences and knowledge and joining the war on prostate cancer to strike yet another blow against this killer. Take this opportunity; it can enrich your life as it has mine.

May you be blessed with good health.

Appendices

Battling The Killer Within

Appendices

What is Prostate Cancer?

Appendix 1

Prostate cancer develops from cells of the prostate gland. Eventually the cancer cells may spread outside the gland to other parts of the body. Most prostate cancers grow very slowly. Autopsy studies show that many elderly men who died of other diseases also had a prostate cancer that neither they nor their doctor were aware of. But some prostate cancers can grow and spread quickly.

The prostate gland is about the size of a walnut and is located in front of the rectum, behind the base of the penis, and under the bladder. It is found only in men, and contains gland cells that produce some of the *seminal fluid*, which protects and nourishes sperm cells.

The prostate surrounds the upper part of the *urethra*, the tube that carries urine and semen out of the penis. Nerves located next to the prostate take part in causing an erection of the penis, and treatments that remove or damage these nerves can cause erectile dysfunction, also known as *impotence*.

Lymph is a clear fluid that contains tissue waste products and immune system cells. *Lymphatic vessels* carry this fluid to *lymph nodes* (small, bean-shaped collections of immune system cells important in fighting infections). Most lymphatic vessels of the prostate lead to pelvic lymph nodes. Cancer cells can enter lymph vessels and spread out along these vessels to reach lymph nodes where they can continue to grow. If prostate cancer cells have multiplied in the pelvic lymph nodes, they are more likely to have spread to other organs of the body as well.

Although several other cell types are found in the prostate, over 99% of prostate cancers develop from glandular cells. The medical term for a cancer that starts in glandular cells is *adenocarcinoma*. Because other types of prostate cancer are so rare, when someone speaks of prostate cancer it is assumed they are referring to a prostatic adenocarcinoma, unless they specifically mention some other cell type.

Prostate-Specific Antigen Blood Test (PSA)

Appendix 2

The American Cancer Society recommends that this blood test to measure PSA (a protein that is made by prostate cells) be offered annually by health care providers to men 50 and older with a life expectancy of at least 10 years, and to younger men who are at high risk of prostate cancer. At this time, the health care provider should also discuss the risks and benefits of early detection and treatment of prostate cancer.

PSA blood test results are reported as *nanograms per milliliter* or *ng/ml*. Results under 4 ng/ml are usually considered normal. The higher the PSA level, the more likely the presence of prostate cancer.

It is important to understand how the PSA blood test is used in early detection of prostate cancer. PSA levels estimate how likely a man is to have prostate cancer but the test does not provide a definite answer. Conditions such as benign prostatic hyperplasia (noncancerous prostate enlargement) and prostatitis (inflammation of the prostate) can cause a borderline or high PSA result.

On the other hand, some men with prostate cancer have negative or borderline PSA results. Certain measures are recommended by many doctors to make PSA testing as accurate as possible. Because ejaculation can cause a temporary increase in blood PSA levels, some doctors suggest that men abstain from sexual activity for two days before testing. Several medications and herbal preparations can lower blood PSA levels. Men having the PSA blood test should tell their doctors if they are taking

Finasteride (Proscar or Propecia), Saw Palmetto (an herb used by some men to treat benign prostate enlargement), or PC-SPES (an herbal mixture that contains Saw Palmetto).

Although the PSA blood test is not perfect, it is the best test currently available for early detection of prostate cancer. Since doctors started using this test, the number of prostate cancers found at an early, curable stage has increased. And since most men have normal test results, they can be reassured that they are unlikely to have prostate cancer, especially if their *digital rectal exam (DRE)* result is also negative.

Men with a high PSA result are advised to have a biopsy, to find out whether or not cancer is present. Test results in the borderline range may cause some confusion. If the DRE result is abnormal, a biopsy is recommended regardless of the PSA levels.

Several new types of PSA tests have recently been suggested as ways to help decide what to do when the usual PSA test result is borderline.

The *percent free PSA test* indicates how much PSA circulates alone in the blood and how much is bound together with other blood proteins. For PSA results in the borderline range, a low percent free PSA means that a prostate cancer is more likely to be present and suggests the need for a biopsy. A recent study found that if men with borderline PSA results had prostate biopsies only when their percent free PSA was 25% or less, about 20% of unnecessary prostate biopsies could be avoided. Although this test is widely used, not all doctors agree whether 25% is the best value to use.

The *PSA velocity* measures how quickly the PSA level rises over a period of time. This is another way to evaluate a man with borderline PSA values. Since the

PSA blood test will need to be repeated the next year to determine PSA velocity, this approach does not provide an immediate answer. A PSA velocity of .75 ng per ml per year is usually considered high. Even when the total PSA value is normal, a high PSA velocity suggests that a cancer may be present and a biopsy should be considered.

The *PSA density (PSAD)* is determined by dividing the PSA number by the prostate volume (its size as measured by transrectal ultrasound). A higher PSAD indicates greater likelihood of cancer.

Age-specific PSA reference ranges are another way to interpret PSA results. It is known that PSA levels are normally higher in older men than in younger men, even in the absence of cancer. For this reason, some doctors have suggested comparing PSA results with results from other men the same age. In practice, a PSA result within the borderline range might be very worrisome in a 50-year-old man but causes less concern in an 80 year old. This is because 80- year-old men without cancer are often bound to have borderline PSA test results. Because cancers missed in older men (when using age-specific PSA reference ranges) may be lethal, this practice has not gained widespread acceptance.

Although the PSA test is used mainly for early detection, it has value in other situations. In men known to have prostate cancer (based on their biopsy result), the PSA test can help predict *prognosis* (outlook). Men with very high PSA results are more likely to have cancer that has spread beyond the prostate and are less likely to be cured or have long-term survival. PSA levels can be used together with clinical examination results and tumor grade to help decide which tests are needed for further evaluation. After surgery or radiation treatment, rising PSA levels can provide an early sign that the cancer is coming back.

Digital Rectal Exam (DRE)

Appendix 3

The American Cancer Society recommends that health care providers offer men who are 50 or older (as well as younger men with high prostate cancer risk) the opportunity to have a procedure called the digital rectal exam (DRE) as part of their annual physical check-up. At this time, the health care provider should also discuss the risks and benefits of early detection and treatment of prostate cancer.

During this examination, a doctor inserts a gloved, lubricated finger into the patient's rectum to feel for any irregular or abnormally firm areas that might be a cancer. The prostate gland is located next to the rectum, and most cancers begin in the part of the gland that can be reached by a rectal exam. While it is uncomfortable, the exam causes no pain and only takes a short time.

Digital rectal examination of the prostate should be performed by health care professionals skilled in recognizing subtle prostate abnormalities such as those of symmetry and consistency, as well as the more classic findings of nodules or hard areas. DRE is less effective than the PSA blood test in finding prostate cancer but can sometimes find cancers in men with normal PSA levels. For this reason, the American Cancer Society guidelines recommend use of both the DRE and PSA blood test for men who choose to undergo testing for early prostate cancer detection. The DRE is also used once a man is known to have prostate cancer, in order to help predict whether the cancer has spread beyond his prostate gland, and to detect cancer that has come back after treatment.

Signs and Symptoms of Prostate Cancer

Appendix 4

Most cases of early prostate cancer cause no symptoms and are found by a PSA blood test and/or DRE. Some prostate cancers may be found because of symptoms such as slowing or weakening of the urinary stream or the need to urinate more often. These symptoms are not specific, and can also be caused by benign diseases of the prostate, such as nodular hyperplasia. Symptoms of advanced prostate cancer include *hematuria* (blood in the urine), *impotence* (difficulty having an erection), and pain in the pelvis, spine, hips, or ribs. These symptoms may also be present with other diseases.

Transrectal Ultrasound (TRUS)

Appendix 5

Transrectal ultrasound (TRUS) uses sound waves to create an image of the prostate on a video screen. Sound waves are released from a small probe placed in the rectum. The sound waves create echoes as they enter the prostate. The same rectal probe detects the echoes that bounce back from the prostate and a computer translates the pattern of echoes into a picture. Because prostate tumors and normal prostate tissue often reflect sound waves differently, this test may be useful in detecting tumors, even those that might be too small or located in areas of the gland that cannot be felt by DRE.

Placing the TRUS probe into the rectum may be temporarily uncomfortable, but the procedure itself is essentially painless. The TRUS examination is done in a doctor's office or outpatient clinic. It usually takes about 10 to 20 minutes.

TRUS is useful when PSA or DRE indicates an abnormality, to guide the biopsy needle into exactly the right area of the prostate. But TRUS is not recommended as a routine test for early detection of prostate cancer.

The Prostate Biopsy

Appendix 6

A biopsy is a surgical procedure in which a sample of tissue is removed for examination under a microscope. A core needle biopsy is the main method used to diagnose prostate cancer. Under transrectal ultrasound guidance a doctor inserts a narrow needle through the wall of the rectum into the area of the prostate gland that appears abnormal or suspicious. The needle then removes a cylinder of tissue, usually about ½ inch long and 1/16 inch across, which is sent to the laboratory to see if cancer is present.

The procedure is usually done in the doctor's office and takes about half an hour. Though the procedure sounds painful, it typically causes little discomfort because a special instrument, called a *biopsy gun*, inserts and removes the needle in a fraction of a second. Several biopsy samples are often taken from different areas of the prostate. Usually six samples are taken (upper, mid, and lower areas of the left and right sides) to get a representative sample of the gland and tell how much of the gland is affected by the cancer. In some cases, as many as eighteen samples may be taken.

Grading the Prostate Cancer

Appendix 7

If cancer is found in a prostate biopsy specimen, it will be *graded* in order to estimate how aggressive it is likely to be (that is how fast it is likely to grow and spread). Grading is done by the pathologist examining the tissue sample taken during the prostate biopsy. Prostate cancers are graded according to how closely they look like normal prostate tissue when viewed under a microscope. The most commonly used prostate cancer grading system is called *the Gleason Grading System.*

This system assigns a *Gleason grade* ranging from 1 through 5 to how much the arrangement of the cancer cells mimics the way normal prostate cells form glands. If the cancer cell clusters resemble the small, regular, evenly spaced glands of normal prostate tissue, a grade of 1 is assigned. If the cancer lacks these features and its cells seem to spread haphazardly through the prostate, it is a grade 5 tumor. Grades 2 through 4 have intermediate features.

Because prostate cancers often have areas with different grades, a grade is assigned to the two areas that make up most of the cancer. These two grades are added together to yield a *Gleason score* (also called the *Gleason sum*) between 2 and 10. Scores of 2 through 4 are often grouped together as low, 5 and 6 are called intermediate, and scores of 7 to 10 are considered high. The higher the score, the more likely that the cancer will grow and spread rapidly, and the worse the patient's *prognosis* (outlook for cure or long-term survival).

Cancers with a high Gleason score are more likely to have already spread beyond the prostate gland at the time they are found. For this reason, the Gleason score (considered together with the blood PSA level and DRE findings) is useful in considering treatment options and selecting additional tests to be done before choosing a treatment.

Prostatic Intraepithelial Neoplasia

Appendix 8

*P*rostatic *intraepithelial neoplasia (PIN)* is a condition in which there are changes in the microscopic appearance (the size, shape, or the rate at which they multiply) of prostate epithelial cells. Older men are more likely to have this condition. PIN is classified as either low grade or high grade. If a person has high-grade PIN, repeat biopsies and PSA tests should be done regularly. PIN *may* lead to the development of prostate cancer. At this time there is no standard treatment for PIN. Studies are being done to determine if treatments used for BPH (benign prostatic hyperplasia) are also effective in treating PIN.

Staging Prostate Cancer

Appendix 9

If the prostate biopsy finds a cancer, more tests are done to find out how far the cancer has spread within the prostate, or nearby tissues or other parts of the body. Staging is the process of gathering information about a cancer from certain examinations and diagnostic tests to determine how widespread it is. The stage of a cancer is the most important factor in choosing treatment options and predicting a patient's outlook for survival. The tests that are done for staging prostate cancer are often based on the man's DRE results, PSA blood test results, and the Gleason score of his cancer.

Physical Examination

The physical exam, especially the digital rectal examination, is an important part of prostate cancer staging. The doctor doing the DRE can tell whether it is likely that the cancer is limited to one side of the prostate, whether it has spread to the other side as well, and if it has probably spread beyond the prostate gland.

Imaging Tests Used for Prostate Cancer Staging

Computed tomography: Commonly known as a CT or CAT scan, this test uses a rotating X-ray beam to create a series of pictures of your body from many angles. A computer combines the information from all these pictures to produce a detailed, cross-sectional image. To highlight details of the CT scan, you may be asked for permission to have a harmless dye injected.

The CT scan may reveal abnormally enlarged lymph nodes. Lymph nodes are a network of bean-sized collections of white blood cells that fight infection. Some prostate cancers spread to nearby lymph nodes, called pelvic lymph nodes. Enlarged pelvic lymph nodes could be a sign of a spreading cancer, or could mean that your body is fighting an infection.

Magnetic resonance imaging (MRI): MRI is like a CT scan except that magnetic fields are used instead of X-rays to create detailed cross-sectional pictures of selected areas of your body. These pictures can show abnormal areas of bones or lymph nodes that suggest cancer may have spread from the prostate.

Radionuclide bone scan: This procedure helps show whether the cancer has spread from the prostate gland to bones. The patient receives an injection of radioactive material. The injection itself is the only uncomfortable part of the entire scanning procedure. The amount of radioactivity involved is low in comparison to the much higher doses used in radiation therapy, and this low level of radiation does not cause any side effects. The radioactive substance is attracted to diseased bone cells throughout the entire skeleton. Areas of diseased bone will be seen on the bone scan image as dense, gray areas, called "hot spots." These areas may suggest metastatic cancer is present, but arthritis or other bone diseases could also cause the same pattern. To distinguish among these conditions, the cancer care team may use other imaging tests or take bone biopsies.

ProstaScint scan: Like the bone scan, the prostascint scan uses low level radioactive material to find cancer that has spread beyond the prostate. Both tests look for areas of the body where the radioactive material collects. But there are several important differences between the two tests.

The radioactive material used for the bone scan collects in areas of damaged bone that may be caused by prostate cancer, other cancers, or benign conditions. The radioactive material for the prostaScint scan is attached to a *monoclonal antibody*, a type of antibody manufactured in the laboratory to recognize and stick to a particular substance. In this case, the antibody specifically recognizes *prostate-specific membrane antigen* (PSMA), a substance found only in normal and cancerous prostate cells.

The advantage of this test is that it detects spread of prostate cancer to bone as well as lymph nodes and other organs, and that it can clearly distinguish prostate cancer from other cancers and benign disorders. Some doctors believe this test is useful in finding metastatic prostate cancer in newly diagnosed patients whose cancer at first appears to be localized to the prostate. The test may also be used when a patient's blood PSA level begins to rise after a period of remission following definitive therapy, but when other tests are not able to find the exact location of the recurrent cancer.

Lymph Node Biopsy

This procedure may be done to find out if cancer has spread from the prostate to nearby lymph nodes. If cancer cells are found in the lymph node biopsy specimen, curative surgery is usually not attempted and other treatment options are considered. There are several options for doing lymph node biopsies.

The surgeon may remove lymph nodes through an incision in the lower part of the abdomen. This is done in the same operation as the planned radical prostatectomy. The nodes are tested in the lab while you are under anesthesia to decide whether the surgeon should continue the radical prostatectomy.

A specially trained radiologist may take a sample of cells from a lymph node by using a technique called *fine needle aspiration (FNA)*. In this procedure, the doctor uses the CT scan image to guide a long, thin needle into the lymph nodes. The syringe attached to the needle takes a small tissue sample from one of the lymph nodes. There is no incision, no scar, and the patient can return home a few hours after the procedure.

A surgeon may use a *laparoscope*, which is a long, slender tube inserted into the abdomen through a very small incision. The laparoscope allows the surgeon to view lymph nodes near the prostate and remove these pelvic lymph nodes using special surgical instruments operated through the laparoscope. Because no large incisions are involved, most people recover fully in only one or two days, and there is virtually no scar left after the operation.

The TNM Staging System

Appendix 10

A *staging system* is a standardized way in which the cancer care team describes the extent to which a cancer has spread. While there are several different staging systems for prostate cancer, the most widely used system in the United States is called the TNM System (also known as the Staging System of the American Joint Committee on Cancer). The TNM System describes the extent of the primary tumor (T stage), the absence or presence of spread to nearby lymph nodes (N stage), and the absence or presence of distant metastasis (M stage).

T stages: There are actually two types of T classifications for prostate cancer. The *clinical stage* is based on digital rectal exam, needle biopsy, and transrectal ultrasound findings. The *pathologic stage* is based on surgical removal and examination of the entire prostate gland, both *seminal vesicles* (two small sacs next to the prostate that store semen) and, in some cases, nearby lymph nodes.

Knowing the clinical stage is important because this information is used in making treatment decisions, such as whether a patient might benefit from surgical removal of the prostate. However, the clinical stage may underestimate the extent of cancer spread, and the pathologic stage determined after surgery is more accurate in predicting the patient's outlook for survival. Men who do not have a radical prostatectomy as their main treatment do not have a pathologic T stage determined.

There are four categories for describing the prostate tumors (T) stage, ranging from T1 to T4.

T1 refers to a tumor that can't be felt during a digital rectal exam, but cancer cells are found in a biopsy specimen. T1 prostate cancers can be further subclassified as T1a, T1b, and T1c.

T2 means that a doctor can feel the prostate cancer by digital rectal exam (DRE) and that the cancer remains within the prostate gland. This category is also subclassified into T2a or T2b. T2a means that the tumor involves only the right or left side of the prostate, but not both sides. If both the left and right sides are involved, it is a T2b cancer.

T3 cancers have spread to the connective tissue next to the prostate and/or to the seminal vesicles, but do not involve any other organs. This group is divided into T3a and T3b. In T3a, the cancer extends outside one or both sides of the prostate, but has not spread to the seminal vesicles. With T3b, the cancer has spread to the seminal vesicles.

T4 means that the cancer has spread to tissues next to the prostate (other than the seminal vesicles), such as the bladders *external sphincter* (muscles that help control urination), the rectum, and/or the wall of the pelvis.

N stages: N0 means that the cancer has not spread to any lymph nodes. N1 indicates spread to one or more regional (nearby) lymph nodes in the pelvis.

M stages: M0 means that the cancer has not metastasized beyond the regional nodes. M1 means metastasis are present in distant (outside of the pelvis) lymph nodes, in bones, or other distant organs such as lungs, liver, or brain.

Stage Grouping

Once a patient's T, N, and M categories have been determined, this information is combined in a process called stage grouping to determine the stage, expressed in Roman numerals from I (the least advanced) to IV (the most advanced stage). The TNM procedures for stage grouping are usually outlined as a table. Some patients find this information useful in understanding their stage and in discussing treatment options with their doctors. Other patients may find this a little overwhelming. The important point is that if you have any questions about your prostate cancer and your treatment options, ask your cancer- care team.

AJCC (TNM) Stage Groupings

Stage I	T1a, N0, M0, low grade or score
Stage II	T1a, N0, M0, intermediate or high grade or score
	T1b, N0, M0, any grade or score
	T1c, N0, M0, any grade or score
	T1, N0, M0, any grade or score
	T2, N0, M0, any grade or score
Stage III	T3, N0, M0, any grade or score
Stage IV	T4, N0, M0, any grade or score
	Any T, N1, M0, any grade or score
	Any T, any N, M1, any grade or score

Prostate Cancer Treatments

Appendix 11

Once the prostate cancer has been diagnosed, graded and staged, there is a lot to consider before choosing a treatment plan.

You may want a second opinion about the best treatment option for your situation, especially if there are several choices available to you. You will want to weigh the benefits of each treatment against its possible side effects or risks. The treatment you choose for prostate cancer should also take into account your age and expected life span, personal preferences and feelings about the side effects associated with each treatment, any other serious health conditions you have, and the stage and grade of your cancer.

Surgery

The two most common prostate operations are radical prostatectomy and transurethral resection of the prostate (TURP).

Radical Prostatecomy: In this operation the entire prostate gland plus some tissue around it is removed. Radical prostatecomy is used most often if the cancer is thought not to have spread outside of the gland.

There are two main types of radical prostatectomy—radical retropubic prostatectomy and radical perineal prostatectomy. In the retropubic operation, the surgeon makes a skin incision in the lower abdomen. The surgeon can remove lymph nodes during this operation through the same incision. A nerve-sparing radical retropubic prostatectomy is a modification of this operation. During this procedure, the surgeon carefully feels the small bundles of nerves on either side of the prostate gland. If it appears that the cancer has not spread to these nerves, the surgeon will not remove them. Because these are the nerves that are needed for erections, leaving them intact lowers (but does not eliminate) the risk of impotence (not being able to have an erection) following surgery.

The radical perineal prostatectomy removes the prostate through an incision in the skin between the scrotum and anus. Nerve-sparing operations are more difficult to perform by this approach and lymph nodes cannot be removed through this incision.

These operations last from 1-1/2 to 4 hours, with the perineal approach taking less time than the retropubic approach. Surgery if followed by an average hospital stay of three days and average time away from work of three to five weeks.

Transurethral resection of the prostate (TURP): In this operation the surgeon removes part of the prostate gland that surrounds the urethra (the tube through which urine exits the bladder). TURP is most often used to treat men with noncancerous enlargement of the prostate called benign prostatic hyperplasia or BPH. The procedure is also used for men with prostate cancer who cannot have a radical prostatectomy because of advanced age or a serious illness (in addition to their prostate cancer).

TURP can be used to relieve symptoms caused by a cancer before other treatments begin. But it is not expected to cure this disease or remove all of the cancer. Cutting through the skin is not done with this surgery. A tool with a small loop of wire on the end is placed insider the prostate through the urethra. Electricity is passed through the wire to heat it and cut the tissue. Either spinal anesthesia or general anesthesia is used.

Cryosurgery: Cryosurgery (also called cryotherapy or cryoablation) is used to treat localized prostate cancer by freezing its cells with a metal probe. Warm saline (saltwater) is circulated through a catheter in the urethra to keep it from freezing. The probe is placed through a skin incision located between the anus and scrotum, and guided into the cancer using transrectal ultrasound.

There are several advantages of cryosurgery. The procedure is less invasive than radical surgery so there is less blood loss, a shorter hospital stay, shorter recovery period, and less pain than radical surgery. The disadvantages are that the long-term effectiveness is unknown since it is a relatively new procedure. Cryosurgery may also have some of the same side effects as other treatments such as radiation therapy and radical surgery. For example, about 82% of patients will experience impotence following cryosurgery. While newer techniques have reduced the occurrence of other side effects, some patients may experience urinary complications such as incontinence, obstruction (blockage of urine flow), a fistula (abnormal passageway between the urethra and rectum), and irritation of the bowel.

Radiation Therapy

Radiation therapy uses high-energy rays (such as gamma rays or X-rays) and particles (such as electrons, protons, or neutrons) to kill cancer cells. Radiation is sometimes used to treat cancer that is still confined within the prostate gland, or has spread to nearby tissue. If the disease is more advanced, radiation may be used to reduce the size of the tumor and to provide relief from present and future symptoms. Radiation usually eliminates the need for surgery. Patients who do not have a good response with radiation therapy may still have surgery ("salvage prostatectomy") at a later date. Two main types of radiation therapy are used—external beam radiation and brachytherapy. There are several forms of these two main types.

External beam radiation therapy: External beam radiation is focused from a source outside the body on the area affected by the cancer. It is much like getting a diagnostic X-ray, but for a longer time. Before treatments start, imaging studies such as CT scans and plain X-rays of the pelvis are done to find the location of the cancer in your body. The radiation team will then make some ink marks on your skin that they will use later as a guide for focusing the radiation in the right area. Patients are usually treated five days per week in an outpatient center over a period of seven or eight weeks, with each treatment lasting a few minutes. The procedure itself is painless.

There are two new forms of external beam radiation that appear promising in increasing the success rate and reducing side effects. Three-dimensional conformal radiation therapy uses sophisticated computers to very precisely map the location of the cancer within the prostate. The patient is fitted with a plastic mold resembling a body cast to keep him still so that the radiation can be more accurately aimed. Radiation beams are then aimed from several directions.

A related technique, conformal proton beam radiation therapy, uses a similar approach to focusing radiation on the cancer. But instead of using X-rays, this technique uses proton beams. Protons are parts of atoms that cause little damage to tissues they pass through but are very effective in killing cells at the end of their path. This means that proton beam radiation may be able to deliver more radiation to the cancer while reducing side effects of nearby normal tissues.

Brachytherapy (internal radiation therapy): Internal radiation therapy, or brachytherapy uses small radioactive pellets (each about the size of a grain of rice) that are directly implanted (permanently or temporarily) into the prostate. Imaging tests such as transrectal ultrasound, CT scans, or MRI are used to accurately guide placement of the radioactive material.

The radioactive materials (isotopes such as iodine 125 or palladium 103) are placed inside thin needles, which are inserted through the skin of the perineum (area between the scrotum and anus) into the prostate. The permanent pellets, which are sometimes called seeds, give off radiation for weeks or months. Because they are so small, their presence causes little discomfort and they are simply left in place after their radioactive material is used up. Alternatively, needles containing more radioactive material can be placed for less than a day. This approach is called high dose rate brachytherapy. For about a week following insertion of the needles, patients may have some pain in the perineal area and may have red-brown discoloration of their urine.

Strontium 89: Strontium 89 (Metastron) is a radioactive substance that is used for treatment of bone pain caused by metastatic prostate cancer. It is injected into a vein and is attracted to areas of bone containing cancer. The radiation given off by the Strontium 89 kills the cancer cells, and relieves the pain caused by bone metastasis. About 80% of prostate cancer patients with painful bone metastasis are helped by this treatment. If prostate cancer has spread to many bones, this approach is much better than trying to aim external beam radiation at each affected bone. In some cases, Strontium 89 is used together with external beam radiation aimed at the most painful bone metastasis.

Hormone Therapy

This treatment is often used for patients whose prostate cancer has spread to other parts of the body or has come back after treatment. Most evidence shows that hormone therapy works better if it is started as early as possible after the cancer has reached an advanced stage. The goal of hormone therapy is to lower levels of the male hormones, androgens. The main androgen is called testosterone. Androgens are produced mainly in the testicles and cause prostate cancer cells to grow. Lowering androgen levels can make prostate cancers shrink or grow more slowly. But hormone therapy does not cure the cancer. There are several methods used for hormone therapy.

Orchiectomy: This operation removes the testicles. Although it is a surgical treatment, orchiectomy is considered a hormonal therapy because it works by removing the main source of male hormones. Orchiectomy lowers androgen levels and can temporarily prevent or reduce growth of most prostate cancers.

Luteinizing hormone-releasing hormone (LHRH) analogs: These drugs decrease the amount of testosterone produced by a man's testicles. LHRH analogs (also called LHRH agonists) are injected either monthly or every three months at the doctor's office or at the oncology center. These drugs can lower the level of testosterone as effectively as surgical removal of the testicles. The two LHRH analogs currently available in the United States are leuprolide (Lupron), and goserelin (Zoladex).

Anti-androgens: Even after orchiectomy or during treatment with LHRH analogs, a small amount of androgen is still produced by the adrenal glands. Anti-androgens block the body's ability to use androgens.

Drugs of this type, such as flutamide (Eulexin) and bicalutamide (Casodex) and nilutamide (Nilandron), are taken as pills, once or three times a day. Anti-androgens are often used in combination with orchiectomy or LHRH analogs. This combination is called total androgen blockade. Early studies suggested that combination therapy might be more effective than LHRH analogs or orchiectomy alone. Larger studies, though, found that the combination isn't really much better than treatment with orchiectomy or LHRH analogs. Some doctors may still prefer to use both together. Others may recommend orchiectomy or LHRH agonists first and then add the anti-androgens if the initial treatment isn't effective enough.

Other hormonal drugs: Diethylstilbestrol (DES), a drug chemically related to the female hormone, estrogen, was once the main form of hormonal therapy for men with prostate cancer. Because of its side effects (which include heart disease and breast enlargement), DES has been mostly replaced by LHRH analogs and anti-androgens.

Other hormonal drugs, megestrol acetate (Megace), and medroxyprogesterone (Depo-Provera), are sometimes used if "first-line" hormonal treatments lose effectiveness. Ketoconazole (Nizoral), first used for treating fungal infections and later found to also work as an anti-androgen, is another drug for "second line" hormonal therapy.

Nearly all prostate cancers treated with hormonal therapy eventually become resistant to this treatment over a period of months or years. Some doctors believe that constant exposure to hormonal drugs might promote resistance, and recommend intermittent treatment with these drugs as an alternative. With intermittent therapy, hormonal drugs are stopped after a man's blood PSA level drops to a very low level and remains stable for a while. If the PSA level begins to rise, the drugs are started again.

Adjuvant hormonal therapy: Hormonal therapy is usually used in men known to have metastatic prostate cancer. Some researchers are currently testing whether adjuvant hormonal therapy (started after radiation or surgery in men without evidence of metastasis) or neoadjuvant hormonal therapy (given before radiation or surgery) will improve survival. The answers to these questions are not yet known.

Chemotherapy

Chemotherapy is used for patients whose prostate cancer has spread outside of the prostate gland and for whom hormone therapy has failed. This treatment is not expected to destroy all the cancer cells, but it may slow tumor growth and reduce pain. Chemotherapy is not recommended as a treatment for men with early prostate cancer.

Chemotherapy uses anticancer drugs that are injection into a vein or muscle, or are taken by mouth. These drugs kill cancer cells, but they also damage some normal cells. The doctor must maintain a delicate balance of chemotherapy doses, making them strong enough to kill the cancer cells but not strong enough to destroy many health cells.

Sometimes, hospitalization may be needed to monitor the treatment and to control its side effects. Some of the chemotherapy drugs used in treating prostate cancer that has returned or continued to grow and spread after treatment with hormonal therapy include doxorubicin (Adriamycin), estramustine, etoposide, mitoxantrone, vinblastine, and paclitaxel. Two or more drugs are often given together to reduce the likelihood of the cancer cells becoming resistant to chemotherapy.

Small cell carcinoma is a rare type of prostate cancer that is more likely to respond to chemotherapy than to hormonal therapy. Small cell carcinoma develops more often in the lungs than in the prostate. Since small cell lung cancer often responds to chemotherapy with cisplatin and etoposide, these drugs are recommended for treating small cell cancers that develop in the prostate.

Expectant Therapy (Watching and Waiting)

For some patients with prostate cancer, the best choice may be expectant therapy with no immediate active treatment. Expectant therapy is also called watching and waiting, watchful waiting, observation, or deferred therapy. Watching and waiting may be recommended if a cancer is not causing any symptoms, is expected to grow very slowly, and is small and contained within one area of the prostate.

This approach is particularly suited for men who are elderly or have other serious health problems. Because prostate cancer often spreads very slowly, many older men who have the disease never need any treatment. Some other men choose watchful waiting because, in their view, the side effects of aggressive treatments outweigh their benefits. Expectant therapy does not mean that a man receives no medical care or follow-up. Rather, his cancer is regularly and carefully observed and monitored. Usually this approach includes a PSA blood test and digital rectal exam every six months, plus a yearly transrectal ultrasound-guided biopsy of the prostate. If a man develops bothersome symptoms or his cancer begins to grow more quickly, decisions about active treatment can be reconsidered.

Prostate Cancer in the United States*
by Race and Ethnicity
1990–200

Appendix 12

Incidence

Race/Ethnicity	Rate
Black	272.1
White	164.3
Hispanic	137.2
Asian/Pacific Islander	100.0
American Indian	53.6

Mortality

Race/Ethnicity	Rate
Black	73.0
White	30.2
Hispanic	24.1
American Indian	21.9
Asian/Pacific Islander	13.9

*Per 100,000 age-adjusted to the 2000 US standard populations.

Prostate Cancer Death Rates*
by Country, 2000

Appendix 13

Highest Death Rate

Rank	Country	Rate
1.	Trinidad & Tobago	32.3
2.	Sweden	27.3
3.	Norway	26.2
4.	Denmark	23.1
5.	Cuba	22.5
6.	Ireland	21.6
7.	New Zealand	21.2
8.	Netherlands	20.0
9.	Chile	19.9
10.	France	19.2
•		
•		
•		
18	United States	17.9

*Death Rates per 100,000

The Atlanta Hope Lodge

Appendix 14

In 1991, the American Cancer Society volunteers and staff conceived the idea of building a Hope Lodge in Georgia. After several studies were conducted, Atlanta was chosen as the site for the facility, due in large part to the increasing number of patients who were travelling to Atlanta for treatment. Atlanta's Hope Lodge is modeled after the other Hope Lodges throughout the country.

In July 1994, Winn-Dixie Stores Foundation and the employees of Winn-Dixie in Atlanta pledged $1 million to launch the campaign, showing an early commitment to the vision of Hope Lodge.

Peter Candler, an American Cancer Society volunteer, led the Hope Lodge project in Atlanta.

In May 1995, Carl Swearingen, another American Cancer Society volunteer, was recruited to raise the funds needed to build the Hope Lodge. The original fundraising goal of $5.3 million was later increased to $5.8 million, so that several additional suites could be built, bringing the total to 34 suites. The fundraising campaign continued for several years as volunteers and staff members contacted companies, foundations, and individuals, requesting their support.

In April 1997 the American Cancer Society broke ground for the Hope Lodge on land that had been donated by the Robert W. Woodruff Health Sciences Center of Emory University.

In February 1998, victory was declared. The campaign was a huge success, raising over $5.8 million. Carl Swearingen announced, "This campaign is a fantastic reflection of the commitment by individuals, businesses, and foundations to those needing a home during cancer treatment."

On June 1, 1998, the door to the American Cancer Society Winn-Dixie Hope Lodge was opened at a special ceremony honoring the volunteers and donors who helped make the dream a reality.

In June 1998, the first cancer patients and their families entered the lodge to find sanctuary, rest, support, and comfort.

Other Hope Lodges:

1. Hope Lodge Birmingham, Alabama
2. Winn-Dixie Hope Lodge, Gainesville, Florida
3. Winn-Dixie Hope Lodge, Miami, Florida
4. Hope Lodge Tampa, Florida
5. Hope Lodge Baltimore, Maryland
6. Hope Lodge Worcester, Massachusetts
7. Hope Lodge Rochester, Minnesota
8. Hope Lodge Kansas City, Missouri
9. Hope Lodge St. Louis, Missouri
10. Hope Lodge Buffalo, New York
11. Hope Lodge Rochester, New York
12. Hope Lodge Greenville, North Carolina
13. Hope Lodge Cincinnati, Ohio
14. Hope Lodge Cleveland, Ohio
15. Hope Lodge Hershey, Pennsylvania
16. Hope Lodge Charleston, South Carolina
17. Hope Lodge Nashville, Tennessee
18. Hope Lodge Burlington, Vermont
19. Hope Lodge Marshfield, Wisconsin
20. Hope Lodge San Juan, Puerto Rico

The American Cancer Society

Appendix 15

In 1913, ten physicians and five laymen founded the American Society for the Control of Cancer. Its stated purpose was to disseminate knowledge about the symptoms, treatment, and prevention of cancer; to investigate conditions under which cancer was found; and to compile statistics about cancer. Later renamed the American Cancer Society, Inc., the organization now consists of more than 2 million volunteers working to conquer cancer.

Organization: The American Cancer Society, Inc., consists of a National Society with chartered divisions throughout the country, and approximately 3,400 units.

The National Society: A national assembly provides basic representation from the divisions and additional representation on the basis of population. The assembly elects a volunteer board of directors, establishes organizational goals, ensures management accountability, and provides stewardship of donated funds. The National Society is responsible for overall planning and coordination of the Society's cancer control activities in prevention, detection, and the enhancement of the quality of life to cancer patients and their families. The National Society also provides technical help and materials for divisions and units, and administers programs of research, medical grants, and clinical fellowships.

The Divisions: These are governed by volunteer members of Division Boards of Directors both medical and lay throughout the US and Puerto Rico.

The Units: Units are organized to deliver cancer control programs in communities throughout the United States. They are led by thousands of local volunteers who direct the activities and programs of the Society at the community level.

National Comprehensive Cancer Network (NCCN) Member Institutions

Appendix 16

City of Hope National Medical Center

Dana-Farber Cancer Institute

Fox Chase Cancer Center

Fred Hutchinson Cancer Research Center

H. Lee Moffitt Cancer Center & Research Institute at the University of South Florida

Huntsman Cancer Institute at the University of Utah

James Cancer Hospital and Solove Research Institute at the Ohio State University

Johns Hopkins Oncology Center

Memorial Sloan-Kettering Cancer Center

Robert H. Lurie Comprehensive Cancer Center of Northwestern University

Roswell Park Cancer Institute

St. Jude Children's Research Hospital

UCSF Stanford Health Care

University of Texas M.D. Anderson Cancer Center

❧ Thomas A Farrington

University of Alabama at Birmingham Comprehensive
Cancer Center

University of Michigan Comprehensive Cancer Center

UNMC/Eppley Cancer Center at the University of
Nebraska Medical Center

ProstRicision® at Radiotherapy Clinics of Georgia

Appendix 17

The physicians of Radiotherapy Clinics of Georgia in Atlanta have specialized in the treatment of prostate cancer since 1977, beginning the retropubic (open) implantation. When it became apparent in 1979 that the old style retropubic technique was ineffective in curing prostate cancer, Dr. Frank Critz, founder of the clinic, began development of simultaneous irradiation, that is, prostate implant, followed by conformal external irradiation. During the next 5 years the technique was refined, and in 1984 RCOG began a formal study of simultaneous irradiation which continues to this day.

In 1992, RCOG changed from the retropublic technique to the transperineal ultrasound guided technique. With the improved seed distribution allowed by the transperineal technique, RCOG was able to double the dose of radiation given to the prostate with a greater margin of safety than could be achieved with the open technique.

While the approach of simultaneous irradiation, performing the implant first then using the seeds as a target for conformal external beam irradiation, made logical sense, it was when PSA was made available for clinical use in 1987 that its true value became apparent. Even in the 1990's, most physicians believed that as long as the PSA was within the normal range after radiotherapy, up to 4 ng/ml, the patient was cancer free. However, Dr. Critz noted early on that men treated with simultaneous irradiation achieved PSAs not just in the normal range, but they achieved undetectable levels, the same as disease-free men achieve after surgery. Even more importantly, the overwhelming majority of men who achieved these undetectable levels remained cancer-free.

Dr. Critz discovery was of immense practical importance. Because there are so many ways to treat prostate cancer, with all doctors claiming their treatment to be best, what men have needed to know is how to evaluate the reported results of treatment. How can a man determine how effective any type of prostate cancer treatment really is? For radical prostatectomy, it is easy: men must achieve and maintain an undetectable PSA, PSA 0.2 ng/ml, for 10 or more years of treatment.

With radiotherapy, though, it is not so easy—even today doctors simply cannot seem to agree on how to define success after radiation. They call success achievement of a PSA nadir less than 4 ng/ml, 2 ng/ml, 1.5 ng.ml, 1 ng/ml or, without three consecutive rises of the PSA (ASTRO definition).

ProstRcision®

ProstRcision® (pronounced PROS-ter-ci-shun) means excision of the prostate by irradiation. In concept, this is similar to removal of the prostate by a radical prostatectomy, but no cutting is involved, so the muscles that control urination are not removed, and the sex nerves are usually not affected. Moreover, the cure rates for the ProstRcision treatment are at least as good as those published for radical prostatectomies.

ProstRcision is founded on logical integration of two separate methods of radiation.

The first step in ProstRcision is the implantation of radioactive I-125 seeds into the prostate. These iodine seeds are tiny metal capsules, 1/5 of an inch long and thin like pencil lead.) The I-125 seeds are implanted into the prostate through an ultrasound-guided transperineal implant technique. This minor surgical procedure is performed in an operating room.

Three weeks following the I-125 seed implant and while the seeds are producing radiation (I-125 has a two-month half-life), conformal beam radiation from a linear accelerator is delivered to the implanted prostate and seminal vesicles.

ProstRcision logically integrates both forms of radiation, the I-125 seed implants and the conformal beam radiation, and utilizes each method to compensate for the ineffectiveness of the other by:

1. Radiation dose intensification through radiation synergy By performing the I-125 implant first and starting conformal beam radiation three weeks later, both normal cells and cancer cells inside the capsule are irradiated simultaneously. Simultaneous radiation produces a synergistic effect, which intensifies the radiation dose *inside* the prostate where most cancer cells are located.

2. Microscopic capsule penetration cancer treatment Microscopic capsule penetration cancer cells, located *outside* the prostate capsule and left untreated by seed implantation alone, are treated by the conformal beam radiation part of ProstRcision.

3. Precision targeting The metal seeds are used as a target for precision conformal beam radiation, which eliminates unnecessary radiation to the adjacent bladder and rectum.

CS Thomas A Farrington

ProstRcision, through the principal of logical integration, effectively treats Stages T1, T2 and T3 prostate cancer. Because cancer cells inside the prostate gland and those that have microscopically penetrated outside the capsule are both effectively treated, ProstRcision eliminates the guesswork about the location and extent of prostate cancer.

The RCOG web site address is www.rcog.net.

RCOG Cure Rate Data

Pre Treatment PSA Groups (ng/ml	10- Year Cure Rates with ProstRcision (% with PSA nadir .02 ng/ml or less)
4.0 or less	96%
4.1 – 10.0	90%
10.1 – 20.0	73%
More than 2.0	71%
Overall	85%

RCOG – John Hopkins Comparison

Institution	Method	10-Year Cure (% with PSA 0.2 or less)
Johns Hopkins	Radical Prostatectomy	80% (overall)
RCOG	RrostRcision	85% (overall)

Partin Table

PSA (ng/ml)	Chance of Microsopic Capsule Penetration
Up to 4.0	10 – 72%
4.1 – 10.0	20 – 87%
101 – 20.0	38 – 94%

Prostate Health Education Network, Inc. (PHEN)
Appendix 18

The Prostate Health Education Network, Inc. was founded in 2003 by Thomas A. Farrington, a prostate cancer survivor and author of *Battling the Killer Within* and *Battling the Killer Within and Winning.*

PHEN is a 501(c)(3) non-profit corporation focusing on the education and awareness needs of African American men. PHEN is also working to highlight and help eliminate the African American prostate cancer disparity through increased visibility and mobilizing resources.

PHEN's activities include:

- Public events to heighten prostate health awareness,
- Seminars and workshops to educate men about their risk, early detection guidelines and treatment options,
- Providing online information via its web portal,
- Screenings
- Establishing and facilitating prostate cancer support groups

For more information visit the PHEN website: www.ProstateHealthEd.org

Personal Prostate Health Management Guide
(Use this guide in consultation with your doctor)
Appendix 19

I. Your Risk Assessment

Risk Factors *(Check all that apply)*

(a) ☐ African American or Sub Saharan African Descent

(b) ☐ Father Diagnosed with Prostate Cancer

(c) ☐ Brother, Grandfather or other close relative Diagnosed with Prostate Cancer

✓ If you checked (a), you are at high risk
✓ If you checked (b), you are at high risk
✓ If you checked (c), you are at high risk
✓ If you checked any combination, you are at high risk plus
✓ If you checked (a), (b) and (c), you are at an even higher risk
✓ If you did not check any of the above, you are not considered at high risk

Your Risk Profile *(Please check)*

☐ Not at High Risk   ☐ High Risk
☐ High Risk Plus

II. Prostate Cancer Early Detection Guidelines: *

- The prostate specific antigen (PSA) test and the digital rectal exam (DRE) should be offered annually beginning at age 50 to men who have a life expectancy of at least 10 years.
- Men at high risk should begin testing at age 45.
- Men with multiple first degree relatives with prostate cancer could begin screening at age 40.
- Physicians should provide information to patients about   benefits and limitations of testing so that patients can make informed decisions.
- Men who request to be tested should not be denied testing.
- Men who request the physician to make the decision for them should be screened.

Adapted from American Cancer Society Guidelines

III. PSA Test Record

	Date	Age	PSA Level	Change**
Base*				
Test 1				
Test 2				
Test 3				
Test 4				
Test 5				
Test 6				
Test 7				

	Date	Age	PSA Level	Change**
Test 8				
Test 9				
Test 10				
Test 11				
Test 12				
Test 13				
Test 14				
Test 15				
Test 16				
Test 17				
Test 18				
Test 19				
Test 20				

*Record your PSA test records for the prior three years, if available, using the first of those years as the base.

**Change is the difference from the prior test–an increase is considered your PSA velocity.

IV. Biopsy Record

If you have been required to get a prostate gland biopsy, complete the following:

1. Year_____ Age_____ PSA____

Biopsy Results:
☐ non cancerous
☐ cancerous ☐ other_____

If Cancerous:
- Gleason score____
- Clinical stage____
- Cancer present in____biopsy samples of___

2. Year_____ Age_____ PSA____

Biopsy Results:
☐ non cancerous
☐ cancerous ☐ other_____

If Cancerous:
- Gleason score____
- Clinical stage____
- Cancer present in____biopsy samples of___

3. Year_____ Age_____ PSA____

Biopsy Results:
☐ non cancerous
☐ cancerous ☐ other_____

If Cancerous:
- Gleason score____
- Clinical stage____
- Cancer present in____biopsy samples of___

V. Post Treatment PSA

If you are treated for prostate cancer, maintain a record of your PSA levels after treatment to determine if you have been cured, or need further treatment. Have your treatment physician outline the cure standards for your treatment.

Month	PSA
6	
12	
18	
24	
36	
42	
48	
54	
66	
72	
78	
84	
90	
96	
102	
108	
114	
120	

Bibliography

"Annual Report." The American Cancer Society, 1999.

Brink, Susan. "Prostate Dilemmas." *U.S. News and World Report*. May 22, 2000.

Baker, William W. "Prostate Cancer: New I-125 Treatment—Simultaneous Irradiation Superior to Surgery." The Garp Report. Garp Research Corporation. Townsend, MD. September 1999.

"Cancer Facts and Figures: 1998." The American Cancer Society, Atlanta.

"Cancer Facts and Figures: 2000." The American Cancer Society, Atlanta.

"Cancer Facts and Figures: 2001." The American Cancer Society, Atlanta.

Chase, Marilyn. "Drop in Prostate Cancer Deaths Fuels Debate Over PSA Blood Test." *The Wall Street Journal*, April 25, 2000.

Clapp, Larry. "Prostate Health in 90 Days." Carlsbad: Hay House, Inc., 1999.

Critz, Frank A. et al., "Simultaneous Irradiation for Prostate Cancer: Intermediate Results with Modern Techniques." *The Journal of Urology*, September 2000.

"Cancer Facts and Figures: 2004." The American Cancer Socitey, Atlanta, Georgia.

Critz, Frank A. et al., "Post-Treatment PSA < 2 ng/ml
    Defines Disease Freedom After Radiotherapy
    for Prostate Cancer Using   Modern
    Technology." *Urology*, v.59, no.6. December
    1999.

Critz, Frank A. et al., "The Cancer Journal." *Scientific
    America*. v. 4, no. 6. November/December
    1998.

"Facts About Prostate Cancer, The." Radiotherapy
    Clinics of Georgia. Decatur.

Grove, Andy, with reporter associate Bethany McLean.
    "Taking on Prostate Cancer." *Fortune*. May 13,
    1996.

Lewis, James Jr. "The Best Options for Diagnosing and
    Treating Prostate Cancer." Westbury, NY: Health
    Education Literary Publisher, 1999.

"Prostate Cancer Treatment Guidelines for Patients."
    Version I, 1999. National Comprehensive
    Cancer Network and The American Cancer
    Society.

Williams, W. Hamilton et al., "African American Men
    with Prostate Cancer Treated by Simultaneous
    Irradiation." *The Prostate Journal*, v.2, no. 2.
    April 2000.

About the Author

Thomas Alex Farrington is an entrepreneur and business executive with more than 30 years experience in the Information Technology industry. In 1969, He was a founder of Input Output Computer Services, Inc. where he served as president and chairman. This company became an early participant in the evolution of IT professional services. IOCS was recognized with countless awards for its business success, and was cited as one of the nations largest black owned businesses by Black Enterprise magazine for more than ten consecutive years. In 1994, Mr. Farrington founded Farrington Associates, Inc.—an information technology consulting firm located in Waltham, Massachusetts.

Throughout his business career, Mr. Farrington has been involved extensively in industry, civic, community, and political activities. He has been selected to serve, at various levels of leadership within many organizations, receiving countless awards and recognitions for his accomplishments. Mr. Farrington was selected one of "Ten Outstanding Young Leaders of Greater Boston." He served as a senior advisor to Massachusetts Governor Michael Dukakis presidential campaign. He was appointed to the Export/Import Bank Advisory Board by President George H. Bush. He was appointed by President Clinton to the Historically Black College Advisory Board. Massachusetts Governor Jane Swift appointed Mr. Farrington to the Massachusetts Technology Park Corporation.

Mr. Farrington serves as a board member of the Greater Boston Chamber of Commerce, and former trustee of

North Carolina A & T State University, Knoxville College, and the Massachusetts Software Council.

After he had authored *Battling the Killer Within* in 2001, Mr. Farrington made numerous presentations about prostate cancer. In 2003, Mr. Farrington founded the Prostate Health Education Network, Inc., (PHEN) to carry out education and awareness initiatives throughout the United States.

Mr. Farrington is a member of St. John's Baptist Church, the Sigma Pi Phi fraternity and The National Association of Guardsmen.

He received his B.S. degree from North Carolina A & T State University in electrical engineering and attended the Northeastern University Graduate School of Engineering.

Index

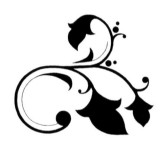

Order Form

To order additional copies, fill out this form and send it along with your check or money order to: FAI, 460 Totten Pond Rd., Waltham, MA 02451

Cost per copy $20.00 plus $3.95 P&H. If shipped to an address in MA, include $1.00 state sales tax.

Ship _____ copies of *Battling the Killer Within and Winning* to:

Name_____

Address:_____

City/State/Zip:_____

All books ordered will be signed by author.

Please tell us how you found out about this book.

☐ Friend   ☐Internet
☐ Book Store   ☐Radio
☐ Newspaper   ☐ Magazine
☐ Other _____